Physical Activity, Fitness, and Health
Consensus Statement

Claude Bouchard, PhD
Laval University
Roy J. Shephard, MD, PhD, DPE
University of Toronto
Thomas Stephens, PhD
Social Epidemiology and Survey Research, Manotick, Ontario

Editors

Human Kinetics Publishers

Library of Congress Cataloging-in-Publication Data

Physical activity, fitness, and health consensus
  statement / [edited by] Claude Bouchard, Roy J. Shephard, Thomas
Stephens.
     p.   cm.
  ISBN 0-87322-470-1
  1. Physical fitness. 2. Exercise. 3. Health. I. Bouchard,
Claude. II. Shephard, Roy J. III. Stephens, Thomas.
  RA781.P563 1993
  613.7--dc20

                                              92-41692
                                                CIP

ISBN: 0-87322-470-1

Developmental Editor: Rodd Whelpley
Assistant Editors: Lisa Sotirelis, Valerie Rose Hall
Copyeditor: Moyra Knight
Proofreader: Dawn Barker
Production Director: Ernie Noa
Typesetting and Layout: Sandra Meier
Text Design: Keith Blomberg
Cover Design: Jack Davis
Cover Photo: David R. Stocklein Photography
Printer: Versa Press

Printed in the United States of America

10 9 8 7 6 5 4 3 2 1

Human Kinetics Publishers
Box 5076, Champaign, IL 61825-5076
1-800-747-4457

Canada Office:
Human Kinetics Publishers
P.O. Box 2503, Windsor, ON N8Y 4S2
1-800-465-7301 (in Canada only)

Europe Office:
Human Kinetics Publishers (Europe) Ltd.
P.O. Box IW14, Leeds LS16 6TR
England
0532-781708

Australia Office:
Human Kinetics Publishers
P.O. Box 80, Kingswood 5062
South Australia
374-0433

Contents

Preface

In May of 1992, the Second International Consensus Symposium on Physical Activity, Fitness, and Health was held in Toronto, Ontario, Canada. This monograph contains the text of the consensus achieved during the 4-day symposium, along with chapters of definitions and information about the organization and conduct of the event. The consensus also focuses on the relationships among physical activity, fitness, and health. The full proceedings of the Consensus Symposium, including the consensus text and the 70 review chapters prepared by the experts who took part in the Consensus Symposium, will be published as *Physical Activity, Fitness, and Health* by Human Kinetics Publishers.

Acknowledgments

The editors of this monograph thank the members of the organizing committees of both the Consensus Symposium and the immediately following International Conference on the topic of physical activity, fitness, and health. The editors are particularly grateful to Dr. Barry McPherson, Wilfrid Laurier University; Dr. Norman Gledhill, York University; Dr. Art Quinney, University of Alberta; and Art Salmon, ParticipACTION, who contributed so much to the development and organization of these events.

The Consensus Symposium Organizing Committee and the Panel of International Advisors

The editors express their gratitude to their colleagues who served on the Consensus Symposium Organizing Committee over a 3-year period, as well as the members of the International Advisory Panel for their contributions to the development and conduct of the Consensus Symposium.

Other Guests and Support Personnel

The editors are also greatly indebted to Ms. Dayle Levine, Executive Assistant, for her support throughout the planning, organization, and execution of the symposium. She played a key role in providing administrative support for the conduct of the meeting. Our thanks also go to Dr. Caroline Davis for organizing the registration and assisting during the consensus process. We also are indebted to Dr. Davis's family for the hospitality extended to all participants during one evening of the symposium. Special thanks also goes to Ms. Veronica Jamnik for her organization of the hospitality and social events and assistance during the consensus meeting. We also especially appreciate Mr. Stan Murray who coordinated on-site transportation.

Finally, we express our gratitude to all volunteers who helped us prepare and complete the meeting. These volunteers were: Janet Bannister, Kelly Broadhurst, Debbie Childs, Michelle Dionne, Tony Doherty, Maria Gurevich, Brandon Hale, Marjorie Hammond, Lyse Jobin, Wendy Keeves, Jodi Liebsman, Denise Mercier, Patricia Murray, Helen Prlic, Marion Reeves, Joe Reischer, Sandra Sawatzky, Ann Marie Vandire, and Lori Wadge.

The Symposium and Conference Organizers gratefully acknowledge the support of the following sponsors and patrons:

Major Sponsors

Ontario Ministry of Tourism and Recreation
Government of Canada, Fitness and Amateur Sport

Additional Sponsors

Air Canada
Canada 125
Canadian Association of Sport Sciences
Canadian Bureau for Active Living
Conners Brewery
Health and Welfare Canada—National Health Research and Development Program
Heart and Stroke Foundation of Canada
Heart and Stroke Foundation of Ontario
Imperial Oil Limited
McDonald's Restaurants of Canada Limited
Medical Research Council of Canada
Merck Frosst Canada Inc.
Molson Breweries of Canada
Ontario Ministry of Citizenship—Office for Seniors' Issues
Ontario Ministry of Health
Ontario Physical and Health Education Association
ParticipACTION
Servier Canada Inc.
Toshiba—Portable Computers and Printers

Patron Universities

Université Laval, Ste-Foy, Québec
University of Alberta, Edmonton, Alberta
Wilfrid Laurier University, Waterloo, Ontario
York University, Downsview, Ontario

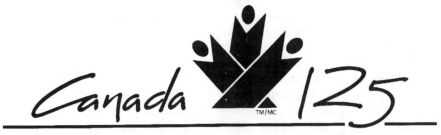

The International Consensus Symposium and The International Conference on Physical Activity, Fitness, and Health were held in conjunction with the celebration of Canada's 125 years of Confederation.

List of Participants

Barbara AINSWORTH
Department of Physical Education
University of North Carolina
CB #8700, Fetzer Gymnasium
Chapel Hill, NC 27599-8700, USA

Per Olof ÅSTRAND
Department of Physiology III
Karolinska Institute
Box 5626
Stockholm S-114-86, Sweden

Richard L. ATKINSON
Department of Internal Medicine
Eastern Virginia Medical School
V.A. Medical Center
Hampton, VA 23667, USA

R. James BARNARD
Department of Kinesiology
University of California at Los Angeles
1804 Life Science
405 Hilgard Avenue
Los Angeles, CA 90024, USA

Oded BAR-OR
Children's Exercise Nutrition Center
Chedoke Hospital
McMaster University
Hamilton, Ontario, Canada L8N 3Z5

Fin BIERING-SØRENSEN
Fysiurgisk Hospital
Rigshospitalet
National University Hospital
25, Havnevej
DK-3100 Hornbæk, Denmark

Steven N. BLAIR
Department of Epidemiology
Institute for Aerobics Research
12330 Preston Road
Dallas, TX 75230, USA

Kari BØ
Norwegian University of Sport and Physical
  Education
P.O. Box 40
KRINGSJÅ 0807, Oslo 8, Norway

Claude BOUCHARD
Physical Activity Sciences Laboratory
Laval University
Ste-Foy, Québec, Canada GlK 7P4

George A. BROOKS
Department of Physical Education
University of California at Berkeley
103 Harmon Gymnasium
Berkeley, CA 94720, USA

Gail E. BUTTERFIELD
Palo Alto Veteran's Administration Medical
  Center
3801 Miranda Avenue
Palo Alto, CA 94304, USA

Marshall W. CARPENTER
Women and Infants Hospital
101 Dudley Street
Providence, RI 02905, USA

Carl J. CASPERSEN
Cardiovascular Health Branch
Centers for Disease Control (K-47)
1600 Clifton Road
Atlanta, GA 30333, USA

Tom CHRISTENSEN
Department of Surgery F
Bispebjerg Hospital
Copenhagen, DK-2400, Denmark

David C. CUMMING
Department of Obstetrics and Gynecology
University of Alberta
1D1 Walter Mackenzie Health Science Center
Edmonton, Alberta, Canada T6G 2R7

Caroline DAVIS
Bethune College
York University
4700 Keele Street
Downsview, Ontario, Canada M3J 1P3

Jerome A. DEMPSEY
Department of Preventive Medicine
University of Wisconsin
504 N. Walnut Street
Madison, WI 53705, USA

Jean-Pierre DESPRÉS
Physical Activity Sciences Laboratory
Laval University
Ste-Foy, Québec, Canada GlK 7P4

Rod K. DISHMAN
Department of Exercise Science
School of Health and Human Performance
University of Georgia
Athens, GA 30602, USA

Barbara DRINKWATER
Department of Medicine
Pacific Medical Center
1200, 12th Avenue S.
Seattle, WA 98144, USA

John V.G.A. DURNIN
Institute of Physiology
The University of Glasgow
Glasgow, G12 8QQ, United Kingdom

Reggie V. EDGERTON
Department of Kinesiology
University of California at Los Angeles
405 Hilgard Avenue
Los Angeles, CA 90024, USA

Randy E. EICHNER
Department of Medicine (EB-271)
University of Oklahoma Health Sciences Center
P.O. Box 26901
Oklahoma City, OK 73190, USA

Robert FAGARD
Department of Medicine
University of Leuven K. U.L.
U.Z. Pellenberg,
Weligerveld I
B-3212 Pellenberg, Belgium

John A. FAULKNER
Department of Physiology
University of Michigan Medical School
7775 Medical Science II - Box 0622
Ann Arbor, MI 48109, USA

Victor FROELICHER
Cardiology Section
VA Medical Center
Stanford University School of Medicine
3801 Miranda Avenue
Palo Alto, CA 94304, USA

Lise GAUVIN
Department of Exercise Science
Concordia University
7141 Sherbrooke Street West
Montréal, Québec, Canada H4B 1R6

Adria GIACCA
Department of Physiology (Rm 3358)
Medical Science Building
University of Toronto
Toronto, Ontario, Canada M5S 1A8

Norman GLEDHILL
Bethune College, Room 343
York University
4700 Keele Street
Downsview, Ontario, Canada M3J 1P3

Andrew P. GOLDBERG
Geriatrics Service (18)
Baltimore Veterans Administration Medical
  Center
3900 Loch Raven Boulevard
Baltimore, MD 21218, USA

Howard J. GREEN
Department of Kinesiology
University of Waterloo
Waterloo, Ontario, Canada N2L 3G1

James M. HAGBERG
Center on Aging
University of Maryland
Room 2304, PERH Building
College Park, MD 20742-2611, USA

Lawrence E. HART
Department of Medicine and Clinical
  Epidemiology
McMaster University Chedoke-McMaster
  Hospital
Box 2000, Station "A"
Hamilton, Ontario, Canada L8N 3Z5

William L. HASKELL
Stanford Center for Research in Disease
  Prevention
Stanford University School of Medicine
730 Welch Road, Suite B
Palo Alto, CA 94304-1583, USA

James O. HILL
Clinical Nutrition Research Unit
Vanderbilt University Hospital
D-4130 MCN
Nashville, TN 37232-2590, USA

Wildor HOLLMANN
Institut für Kreislaufforschung und Sportmedizin
Deutsche Sporthochschule
5000 Köln 41, Carl Diem Weg
Köln, Müngersdorf, Germany

Robert KAMAN
Departments of Physiology, Public Health and
  Preventive Medicine
Texas College of Osteopathic Medicine
3500 Camp Bowie Boulevard
Fort Worth, TX 76107, USA

Harold W. KOHL
Institute for Aerobics Research
12330 Preston Road
Dallas, TX 75230, USA

Daniel M. LANDERS
Exercise and Sport Research Institute
Department of Health and Physical Education
Arizona State University
Tempe, AZ 85287, USA

M. Harold LAUGHLIN
Departments of Veterinary Biomedical Sciences
 and Medical Physiology
University of Missouri
W117-Veterinary Medical Building
Columbia, MO 65211, USA

I-Min LEE
Department of Epidemiology
School of Public Health
Harvard University
677 Huntington Avenue
Boston, MA 02115, USA

Pierre LEFEBVRE
Département de Médecine
Centre Hospitalier Universitaire de Liège
Domaine Universitaire du Sart Tilman
Bloc central +2-B35
B-4000 Liège, Belgique

Arthur S. LEON
Division of Applied Physiology-Nutrition
Division of Epidemiology
School of Public Health
University of Minnesota
Minneapolis, MN 55455, USA

Anne B. LOUCKS
Department of Zoological and Biomedical
 Sciences
Ohio University
Athens, OH 45701-2979, USA

Duncan MacDOUGALL
Department of Physical Education
McMaster University
1280 Main Street West
Hamilton, Ontario, Canada L8S 4K1

Robert M. MALINA
Department of Kinesiology and Health
 Education
University of Texas at Austin
Austin, TX 78712, USA

Edward McAULEY
Department of Kinesiology
University of Illinois at Urbana-Champaign
215 Freer Hall
Champaign, IL 61801, USA

Neil McCARTNEY
Department of Physical Education
McMaster University
1280 Main Street West
Hamilton, Ontario, Canada L8S 4K1

Barry McPHERSON
Faculty of Graduate Studies
Wilfrid Laurier University
75 University Street
Waterloo, Ontario, Canada N2L 3C5

Jere H. MITCHELL
UT Southwestern Medical Center
5323 Harry Hines Boulevard
Dallas, TX 75235, USA

Henry J. MONTOYE
Biodynamics Laboratory
University of Wisconsin-Madison
2000 Observatory Drive
Madison, WI 53706, USA

Sean MOORE
Department of Pathology
McGill University
3775 University Street
Montréal, Québec, Canada H3A 2B4

William P. MORGAN
Sport Psychology Laboratory
University of Wisconsin-Madison
2000 Observatory Drive
Madison, WI 53706, USA

Frank M. MOSES
Gastroenterology Service
Walter Reed Army Medical Center
6900 Georgia Avenue
Washington, DC 20307-5001, USA

Michelle MOTTOLA
Faculty of Kinesiology
The University of Western Ontario
Thames Hall
London, Ontario, Canada N6A 3K7

Eric A. NEWSHOLME
Department of Biochemistry
Merton College
University of Oxford
South Parks Road
Oxford OX1 3QU, United Kingdom

David C. NIEMAN
Department of Health, Leisure and Exercise
 Sciences
Appalachian State University
Boone, NC 28608, USA

Tim D. NOAKES
Department of Physiology
University of Cape Town Medical School
Observatory 7925, South Africa

Pekka OJA
President Urho Kaleva Kekkonen Institute for
    Health Promotion Research
Kaupinpuistonkatu 1
SF-33500 Tampere 50, Finland

Neil OLDRIDGE
Department of Health Sciences
University of Wisconsin-Milwaukee
P.O. Box 413
Milwaukee, WI 53201, USA

Ralph PAFFENBARGER
Department of Health Research and Policy
Stanford University School of Medicine
Stanford, CA 94305-5092, USA

Richard S. PANUSH
Department of Medicine
New Jersey Medical School
Old Short Hills Road
Livingston, NJ 07039, USA

Russell R. PATE
Department of Exercise Science
School of Public Health
University of South Carolina
Columbia, SC 29208, USA

Louis PÉRUSSE
Physical Activity Sciences Laboratory
Laval University
Ste-Foy, Québec, Canada G1K 7P4

Michael J. PLYLEY
School of Physical and Health Education
University of Toronto
320 Huron Street
Toronto, Ontario, Canada M5S 1A1

Janet POLIVY
Department of Psychology
Erindale Campus
University of Toronto
3359 Mississauga Road
Mississauga, Ontario, Canada L5L 1C6

Kenneth E. POWELL
Division of Injury Control
Centers for Disease Control
Mailstop F-36
1600 Clifton Road, N.E.
Atlanta, GA 30333, USA

Art QUINNEY
Faculty of Physical Education and Sports Studies
University of Alberta
Edmonton, Alberta, Canada T6G 2H9

Rainer RAURAMAA
Kuopio Research Institute of Exercise Medicine
Puistokatu 20
70110 Kuopio, Finland

Peter RAVEN
Department of Physiology
Texas College Osteopathic Medicine
3500 Camp Bowie Boulevard
Fort Worth, TX 76107-2690, USA

Elizabeth READY
Faculty of Physical Education and Recreation
    Studies
University of Manitoba
Winnipeg, Manitoba, Canada R3T 2N2

W. Jack REJESKI
Department of Health and Sport Science
Wake Forest University
307 Reynolds Gymnasium, Box 7234
Winston-Salem, NC 27109, USA

Michael J. RENNIE
Department of Anatomy and Physiology
The University of Dundee
Dundee DD1 4HN, Scotland

Erik A. RICHTER
August Krogh Institute
University of Copenhagen
13 Universitetsparken
DK-2100 Copenhagen Õ, Denmark

James F. SALLIS
Department of Psychology
San Diego State University
San Diego, CA 92182, USA

Art SALMON
ParticipACTION
P.O. Box 64
40 Dundas Street West
Toronto, Ontario, Canada M5G 2C2

Mike SHARRATT
Faculty of Applied Health Sciences
University of Waterloo
Waterloo, Ontario, Canada N2L 3G1

Roy J. SHEPHARD
School of Physical and Health Education
University of Toronto
320 Huron Street
Toronto, Ontario, Canada M5S 1A1

James S. SKINNER
Exercise and Sport Research Institute
Arizona State University
Tempe, AZ 85287-0404, USA

Marcia L. STEFANICK
Stanford Center for Research in Disease
    Prevention
Stanford University School of Medicine
730 Welch Road, Suite B
Palo Alto, CA 94304-1583, USA

George STELMACH
Exercise and Sport Science Institute
Arizona State University
Tempe, AZ 85287-0404, USA

Thomas STEPHENS
Social Epidemiology and Survey Research
Box 837, 1118 John Street
Manotick, Ontario, Canada K4M 1A7

John R. SUTTON
Cumberland College of Health Sciences
The University of Sydney, P.O. Box 170
Lidcombe, N.S.W., Australia 2141

Jerry R. THOMAS
Department of Exercise Science and Physical
    Education
Arizona State University
Tempe, AZ 85287-0701, USA

Paul D. THOMPSON
University of Pittsburgh Heart Institute
Montefiore University Hospital
B-Level, South, 3459 Fifth Avenue
Pittsburgh, PA 15213, USA

Charles M. TIPTON
Department of Exercise and Sport Sciences
University of Arizona
Ina E. Gittings Building
Tucson, AZ 85721, USA

Angelo TREMBLAY
Physical Activity Sciences Laboratory
Laval University
Ste-Foy, Québec, Canada G1K 7P4

Arthur C. VAILAS
Biodynamics Laboratory
University of Wisconsin
2000 Observatory Drive
Madison, WI 53706, USA

Mladen VRANIC
Department of Physiology (Rm 3358)
Medical Science Building
University of Toronto
Toronto, Ontario, Canada M5S 1A8

Ilkka M. VUORI
President Urho Kekkonen Institute for Health
    Promotion Research
Kaupinpuistonkatu 1
SF-33500 Tampere 50, Finland

Leonard M. WANKEL
Faculty of Physical Education and Recreation
University of Alberta
E-411 Physical Education Building
Edmonton, Alberta, Canada T6G 2H9

Brian J. WHIPP
Department of Physiology
St-George's Hospital Medical School
University of London
Cranmer Terrace
Tooting
London SW17 ORE, England

Melvin H. WILLIAMS
Human Performance Laboratory
Old Dominion University
Health and Physical Education Building
Norfolk, VA 23529-0196, USA

Jack H. WILMORE
Department of Kinesiology and Health
    Education
The University of Texas at Austin
Austin, TX 78712, USA

Peter D. WOOD
Stanford Center for Research in Disease
    Prevention
Stanford University School of Medicine
730 Welch Road, Suite B
Palo Alto, CA 94304-1583, USA

The Consensus
Document

Chapter 1

Introduction

Canada, and particularly Toronto, has a long-standing tradition with regard to the organization of consensus meetings pertaining to the broad topics of exercise and health. An early initiative was the International Conference on Physical Activity and Cardiovascular Health convened by Roy Shephard in 1966. Toronto was also the site of the 1988 International Consensus Conference on Exercise, Fitness, and Health. In 1992, to coincide with Canada's 125th birthday, two further international meetings were convened in Toronto over a 10-day period. The first of the most recent meetings was the Second International Consensus Symposium on Physical Activity, Fitness, and Health. This monograph is the official publication of the consensus text developed during the symposium. The full proceedings of the Consensus Symposium, including the consensus text and 70 chapters detailing the supportive evidence, are published by Human Kinetics Publishers in a separate publication. The second meeting was a Conference on Physical Activity, Fitness, and Health (the Active Living Conference). The conference was open to all those interested in the areas of program and policy development as it pertains to physical activity, fitness and health. The proceedings of that conference are presented in a separate publication also from Human Kinetics Publishers.

The objectives of the 1992 Second International Consensus Symposium on Physical Activity, Fitness, and Health were as follows:

- To revise and expand the 1988 Consensus Statement from the perspective of the biological, social and behavioral sciences.
- To achieve a better integration of the evidence regarding the respective and interactive contributions to health of regular physical activity and physical fitness.
- To review in greater depth the evidence linking the components in a general model.
- To provide a better description of the effects of growth, gender, aging and social environments upon the basic model.
- To provide a better quantification of the amount of habitual physical activity associated with each outcome (i.e., the dose-response issue).
- For each topic, to identify the type (experimental, epidemiological, clinical), the quality, and the extent of evidence supporting the conclusions.
- To identify in greater detail, and in a more systematic manner, areas of needed research and the most pressing questions to be addressed.
- To contribute to the knowledge base for the 1992 Conference on Active Living.

The Consensus Symposium Organizing Committee

A Consensus Symposium Organizing Committee took responsibility for the planning, the program development, the organization and the conduct of the event. The members of the Committee and their functions were as follows:

Dr. Claude BOUCHARD
Chairperson of the Consensus Symposium Organizing Committee
Université Laval
Ste-Foy, Québec

Dr. Norman GLEDHILL
Chair of Finance Committee
York University
Downsview, Ontario

Ms. Dayle LEVINE
Executive Assistant
York University
Downsview, Ontario

Dr. Barry McPHERSON
President of the Conference and Consensus Symposium Board
Wilfrid Laurier University
Waterloo, Ontario

Dr. Art QUINNEY
Chairperson of Active Living Conference Organizing Committee
University of Alberta
Edmonton, Alberta

Dr. Elizabeth READY
University of Manitoba
Winnipeg, Manitoba

Mr. Art SALMON
Chair of the Site Committee
ParticipACTION
Toronto, Ontario

Dr. Roy J. SHEPHARD
University of Toronto
Toronto, Ontario

Dr. Thomas STEPHENS
Consultant
Manotick, Ontario

The International Advisors

In addition, a panel of seven advisors from five countries assisted the Consensus Symposium Organizing Committee. The members of this International Advisory Panel were:

Dr. Per-Olof ÅSTRAND
Stockholm, Sweden

Dr. Steven N. BLAIR
Dallas, Texas, USA

Dr. Barbara L. DRINKWATER
Vashon, Washington, USA

Dr. Wildor HOLLMANN
Cologne, Germany

Dr. William P. MORGAN
Madison, Wisconsin, USA

Dr. Eric A. NEWSHOLME
Oxford, England

Dr. John SUTTON
Lidcombe, Australia

Planning of the Consensus Symposium

After 18 months and several meetings of the Consensus Symposium Organizing Committee, the preparation of numerous working documents, an extensive literature search, and frequent exchanges with the International Advisors, a total of 72 topics were selected for inclusion in the program.

A bank of names of individuals with expertise on each topic was created, based on the advice of members of the Consensus Symposium Organizing Committee and the International Advisory Panel. For each name on the list, a computer searched all papers published over the last five years, based on the Institute for Scientific Information literature banks. This list was compiled for each of about 600 scientists. The three to five most productive persons for each topic were retained, and a Science Citation Index or Social Science Citation Index study was carried out on each of them, using the services of the Institute for Scientific Information. The citation surveys were undertaken for about 350 scientists. The process yielded a first and second choice of experts for approximately 65 of the 72 topics. Further consultation was needed to identify the most active group of scientists for the remaining topics.

Invitations were issued to one or two experts per topic about 15 months prior to the Consensus Symposium. Each expert was given the following assignments:

- To prepare a two-page draft of the consensus text proposed for the topic at least three months before the meeting.
- To prepare a full paper documenting the research available on the topic, to be delivered before the symposium with the understanding that it would be revised before publication.
- To attend the 4-day Consensus Symposium in Toronto.
- To participate in the development of the final consensus text.

A document describing the model and the key concepts upon which the Consensus Symposium was based (see chapter 2 by Bouchard and Shephard) was distributed to all participants 6 months prior to the meeting. A series of criteria to be used in the evaluation of the available evidence was also distributed to all participants well ahead of the meeting.

The Consensus Development Process

Based on drafts of the 72 consensus proposals, a preliminary consensus text was prepared and revised by the three editors of this publication. After several rounds of corrections and amendments, the preliminary consensus document was made available to all invited participants about one month prior to the meeting. This text served as the basis for the discussion at the Consensus Symposium.

During the Consensus Symposium, the invited experts were divided into eight working groups. These working groups were constituted around clusters of topics determined by affinity of subject matter. In addition to attending plenary sessions, each working group met for 6 to 8 hours per day, reviewing the evidence and amending or rewriting the consensus statement for the topics that had been assigned to that group. A group leader organized the agenda and ensured that discussion proceeded in an orderly manner. In particular, leaders were encouraged to seek input from all participants, to avoid retreating to bland compromise, and to seek consensus but not necessarily unanimity. Administrative and secretarial support was provided to prepare and distribute revised drafts to members of each group. The major themes, the leaders, the invited participants, and the topics discussed by each group are listed here.

Group 1	Topics

ASSESSMENT, DETERMINANTS, AND ADJUVANTS

Group Leader: Neil Oldridge, Milwaukee, USA

Ainsworth, Barbara E.	
Butterfield, Gail E.	Physical activity and nutrition in the context of fitness and health (with A. Tremblay)
Caspersen, Carl J.	Measurement of health status and well being (with K.E. Powell)
Dishman, Rod K.	Determinants of participation in physical activity (with J.F. Sallis)
Gledhill, Norman	
Kaman, Robert	Costs and benefits of an active versus an inactive society (not reviewed by Group 1)
Leon, Arthur S.	Methods of assessing physical activity during leisure and work (with H.J. Montoye)
Montoye, Henry J.	Methods of assessing physical activity during leisure and work (with A.S. Leon)
Oja, Pekka	Laboratory and field tests for assessing health-related fitness (with J.S. Skinner)
Powell, Kenneth E.	Measurement of health status and well being (with C.J. Caspersen)
Sallis, James F.	Determinants of participation in physical activity (with R.K. Dishman)
Skinner, James S.	Laboratory and field tests for assessing health-related fitness (with P. Oja)
Tremblay, Angelo	Physical activity and nutrition in the context of fitness and health (with G.E. Butterfield)
Vuori, Ilkka	Adjuvants to physical activity (with J.H. Wilmore)
Wilmore, Jack H.	Adjuvants to physical activity (with I. Vuori)

Group 2	Topics

HEART AND VASCULAR

Group Leader: Peter Raven, Fort Worth, USA

Barnard, James R.	Physical activity, fitness, and claudication (peripheral vascular disease)
Blair, Steven N.	Physical activity, fitness, and coronary heart disease
Fagard, Robert	Physical activity, fitness, and hypertension (with C.M. Tipton)
Froelicher, Victor F.	Physical activity, fitness, and CHD rehabilitation
Haskell, William	Dose-response issues from a biological perspective (not reviewed by Group 2)
Kohl, Harold W.	Physical activity, fitness, and stroke
Laughlin, M. Harold	Physical activity and the microcirculation
Mitchell, Jere	Cardiovascular adaptation to physical activity (with P. Raven)
Moore, Sean	Physical activity, fitness, and atherosclerosis
Thompson, Paul D.	Risk of exercising: medical risks and sudden death
Tipton, Charles M.	Physical activity, fitness, and hypertension (with R. Fagard)
Rauramaa, Rainer	Physical activity, fibrinolysis, and platelet aggregability

Group 3	Topics

PULMONARY, DIGESTIVE, AND URINARY

Group Leader: Michael J. Plyley, Toronto, Canada

Bø, Kari	Physical activity, fitness, and bladder
Dempsey, Jerome A.	Pulmonary adaptation to physical activity
Eichner, Randy E.	Physical activity and free radicals
Goldberg, Andrew P.	Physical activity, fitness, and kidney diseases
Hart, Lawrence E.	Assessing the level and quality of evidence and identifying research needs (not reviewed by Group 3)
Moses, Frank M.	Physical activity and digestive processes
Noakes, Tim D.	Physical activity and iron metabolism
Quinney, Art	
Whipp, Brian J.	Physical activity, fitness, and chronic lung diseases

Group 4	Topics

METABOLISM

Group Leader: Elizabeth Ready, Winnipeg, Canada

Atkinson, Richard	Physical activity, fitness, and severe obesity
Brooks, George A.	Physical activity and carbohydrate metabolism
Després, Jean-Pierre	Physical activity and adipose tissue
Faulkner, John A.	Physical activity and skeletal muscle (with H.J. Green)
Giacca, Adria	Physical activity, fitness, and Type I diabetes (with M. Vranic)
Green, Howard J.	Physical activity and skeletal muscle (with J.A. Faulkner)
Hill, James O.	Physical activity, fitness, overweight, and moderate obesity
Lefebvre, Pierre	Physical activity, fitness, and Type II diabetes
Rennie, Michael J.	Physical activity and protein metabolism
Richter, Eric A.	Hormonal adaptation to physical activity (with J.R. Sutton)
Stefanic, Marcia L.	Physical activity, lipid metabolism, and lipid transport (with P.D. Wood)
Sutton, John R.	Hormonal adaptation to physical activity (with E.A. Richter)
Vranic, Mladen	Physical activity, fitness, and Type I diabetes (with A. Giacca)
Wood, Peter D.	Physical activity, lipid metabolism, and lipid transport (with M.L. Stefanic)

Group 5	Topics

INFECTION, TRAUMA, AND RISKS

Group Leader: Mike Sharratt, Waterloo, Canada

Biering-Sørensen, Fin	Physical activity, fitness, and back pain
Christensen, Tom	Physical activity, fitness, and recovery from surgery or trauma
Drinkwater, Barbara L.	Physical activity, fitness, and osteoporosis
Lee, I-Min	Physical activity, fitness, and cancer
Newsholme, Eric A.	Physical activity, fitness, immune function, and immune disorders
Nieman, David C.	Physical activity, fitness, and infection

Group 5 (Cont.)	Topics
Panush, Richard S.	Physical activity, fitness, and osteoarthritis
Pate, Russell R.	Risk of exercising: musculoskeletal injuries and recreational vehicle accidents
Shephard, Roy J.	Demography of health-related fitness level within and between populations (reviewed by Group 1)
Vailas, Arthur C.	Physical activity and bone and connective tissue

Group 6	Topics

SOCIAL AND PSYCHOLOGICAL ISSUES

Group Leader: Lise Gauvin, Montréal, Canada

Landers, Daniel M.	Physical activity, fitness, and anxiety
McAuley, Edward	Physical activity and psychosocial outcomes
McPherson, Barry	
Morgan, William P.	Physical activity, fitness, and depression
Polivy, Janet	Physical activity, fitness, and compulsive behaviors
Rejeski, Jack W.	Dose-response issues from a psychosocial perspective
Stephens, Thomas	Demography of participation in physical activity within and between populations (reviewed by Group 1)
Thomas, Jerry R.	Physical activity and intellectual performance
Wankel, Leonard M.	Physical activity and lifestyle behavior
Williams, Melvin H.	Physical activity, fitness, substance misuse and abuse

Group 7	Topics

BRAIN, NERVOUS SYSTEM, AND AGING

Group Leader: Duncan MacDougall, Hamilton, Canada

Åstrand, Per Olof	Physical activity and fitness: evolutionary perspective and trends for the future (not reviewed by Group 7)
Durnin, John	
Edgerton, Reggie V.	Physical activity and peripheral nervous system
Hagberg, James M.	Physical activity, fitness and health, and aging
Hollmann, Wildor	Physical activity and the brain
McCartney, Neil	Physical activity, fitness, and the physically disabled

Group 7 (Cont.)	Topics
Paffenbarger, Ralph	Physical activity, fitness, and quality-adjusted life expectancy (not reviewed by Group 7)
Stelmach, George	Physical activity and perceptual and sensory mechanisms

Group 8	Topics

REPRODUCTIVE HEALTH AND GROWTH

Group Leader: Michelle Mottola, London, Canada

Bar-Or, Oded	Childhood and adolescent physical activity and fitness and adult risk profile
Carpenter, Marshall W.	Physical activity, fitness, and health of the pregnant mother and fetus
Cumming, David C.	Physical activity, fitness, and reproductive health in men
Loucks, Anne B.	Physical activity, fitness, and menstrual cycles
Malina, Robert M.	Physical activity, fitness, and growth and development
Pérusse, Louis	Heredity, activity level, fitness, and health (with C. Bouchard) (not reviewed by Group 8)

The working groups were instructed to produce the most valid and complete consensus statement for each topic that had been assigned to them based on the available scientific evidence after taking into account the quality of that evidence. The consensus statement was to be prepared in terms of current status of knowledge and important research questions to be addressed. The consensus document is included in chapters 4 to 10 of the present publication. Chapter 11 was not a part of the consensus development process. The four sections included in that particular chapter were reviewed by the editors of the present publication and by several external reviewers.

It is important to recognize that each invited expert reviewed critically and approved the consensus text only for the topics that were on the agenda of his or her particular working group.

However, the full consensus document was not reviewed and approved by all the experts taking part in the Consensus Symposium. The three editors assumed responsibility for the final text, paying attention to overall organization of text, redundancies, terminology, grammar, and spelling.

Although this consensus statement has not been reviewed in its entirety by all the symposium attendees, each section represents the collective views of several scientists who spent many hours reviewing and debating the evidence assembled by one of the working group members over the previous year. Thus, the editors feel confident that this statement represents the informed opinion of the most active scientists in each area concerning the relationships of physical activity, fitness and health.

Chapter 2

Physical Activity, Fitness, and Health: The Model and Key Concepts

Claude Bouchard
Roy J. Shephard

This document describes the basic model used at the Consensus Symposium to specify the relationships between physical activity, health-related fitness, and health.

An Overview of the Model

The subject matter has been approached on the assumption that the relationships between the levels of physical activity, health-related fitness, and health are complex (see Figure 2.1). The model specifies that habitual physical activity can influence fitness, which in turn may modify the level of habitual physical activity. For instance, with increasing fitness, people tend to become more active while the fittest individuals tend to be the most active. The model also specifies that fitness is related to health in a reciprocal manner. That is, fitness not only influences health, but health status also influences both habitual physical activity level and fitness level.

Other factors are associated with individual differences in health status. Likewise, the level of fitness is not determined entirely by an individual's level of habitual physical activity. Other lifestyle behaviors, physical and social environmental conditions, personal attributes, and genetic characteristics also affect the major components of the basic model and determine their interrelationships. The program content of the Consensus Symposium was planned to explore the relationships outlined in this figure.

Physical Activity

An active individual values physical activity as an important part of her or his total life experience and seeks to integrate such activity into daily routines and leisure pursuits throughout all aspects and stages of life. Physical activity comprises any body movement produced by the skeletal muscles that results in a substantial increase over the resting energy expenditure. Under this broad rubric, we consider active physical leisure, exercise, sport, occupational work and chores, together with other factors modifying the total daily energy expenditure. From the viewpoints of fitness and health, all determinants of human energy expenditure merit careful consideration.

Leisure-Time Physical Activity

In most developed societies, after completion of work, travelling, domestic chores and personal hygiene, the average person has 3-4 hours of "free," leisure, or discretionary time per day (32,68). However, there is wide inter-individual variation, depending in part upon such personal circumstances as the duration of paid work, the division of labor in the home (women often accepting more domestic duties than men), the need for self-sufficiency activities (greater in those with a limited income), daily travel time (significant for many people who live in large metropolitan areas), and the number and age of dependents.

Leisure-time physical activity is an activity undertaken in the individual's discretionary time that leads to any substantial increase in the total daily energy expenditure. The element of personal choice is inherent to the definition. Activity is selected on the basis of personal needs and interests. In some instances, the motivation will be an improvement of health and/or fitness, and the pattern of activity undertaken will be consonant with this objective. But there are many other possible motivations (21,40,61) including aesthetic (pursuit of a designed

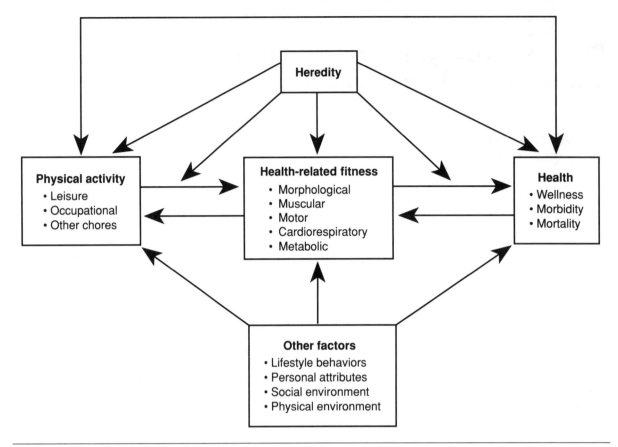

Figure 2.1 A model describing the relationships among habitual physical activity, health-related fitness, and health status.

body type or an appreciation of the beauty of movement), ascetic (the setting of a personal physical challenge), thrill of fast movement and physical danger, chance and competition, social contacts, fun, mental arousal, relaxation and detente, and even addiction to endogenous opioids.

Exercise

Exercise is a form of leisure-time physical activity that is usually performed on a repeated basis over an extended period of time (exercise training) with a specific external objective such as the improvement of fitness, physical performance, or health. When prescribed by a physician or exercise specialist, the optimum regimen advised typically covers the recommended mode, intensity, frequency, and duration of such activity (1).

Mode

The *mode* of exercise covers not only the type of activity to be performed (for instance, fast walking, jogging, or swimming), but also the *temporal pattern*

of activity that is recommended (that is, continuous or intermittent activity), with a detailed specification of the duration of exercise and rest periods in the case of intermittent activity bouts. The issues of *intensity*, *frequency* and *duration* of exercise are therefore of considerable importance to prescription and activity assessment.

Intensity

The intensity of exercise can be expressed in either absolute or relative terms. The absolute intensity (for example, 20 kJ/min) is frequently used when classifying participants in occupational and epidemiological studies. Alternatively, absolute data may be expressed as a multiple of the individual's basal metabolic rate, thereby minimizing differences of energy expenditure between individuals due to differing body mass. Relative intensity is a percentage of the individual's maximal aerobic power output, maximal oxygen intake, or maximal heart rate. If due allowance is made for the influence of age on maximal aerobic power, the absolute and relative approaches can be reconciled (see Table 2.1).

Table 2.1   A Characterization of the Intensity of Leisure Activity in Relation to the Subject's Age*

Categorization	Relative intensity (% $\dot{V}O_2$max)	Absolute intensity (METs)			
		Young	Middle-aged	Old	Very old
Rest	<10	1.0	1.0	1.0	1.0
Light	<35	<4.5	<3.5	<2.5	<1.5
Fairly light	<50	<6.5	<5.0	<3.5	<2.0
Moderate	<70	<9.0	<7.0	<5.0	<2.8
Heavy	>70	>9.0	>7.0	>5.0	>2.8
Maximal	100	13.0	10.0	7.0	4.0

*From reference 10. Note that currently there is a trend to prescribe fairly light and moderate intensity activities rather than heavier intensity activities.

Individual self-reports of activity participation can be categorized in terms of the intensity scales for occupation and leisure activity (see Table 2.2), taking account of both the pursuit and the frequency of its repetition. For instance, occasional swimming is likely to involve less intense activity than participation in a regular swimming program, and this in turn will involve less intense exercise than formal preparation for a major swimming competition.

Frequency

The frequency of leisure activity is normally reported as the number of sessions undertaken in a typical week, although occasional surveys have recorded less frequent participation, for example monthly. One important source of difficulty when reporting frequency is that many leisure activities are seasonal in nature. The epidemiologist thus finds it helpful to ask the frequency of participation during the past week or month and to overcome seasonal variations by questioning different individuals at different times during the year. Extend-

ing the reporting period to a full year is another approach but may suffer from recall problems.

Duration

The duration of an individual exercise session is usually reported in minutes or in hours. It is important that only the period of actual physical activity be considered, omitting travel, socializing, and preparations for participation (62). As with frequency, typical and usual duration is generally recorded although this may vary greatly.

Sport

In North America, sport implies a form of physical activity that involves competition. However, in Europe, the term sport may also embrace exercise and recreation (as in the UNESCO "Sport for All" movement, 51). There is some discussion as to whether required school programs and professional activities should be included in the category of sport because the important element of the participant's choice is then largely eliminated.

Table 2.2   Intensity of Occupational Work*

Intensity	Energy expenditure
Sedentary	<8.4 kJ/min
Light	8.4 - 14.7 kJ/min
Moderate	14.7 - 20.9 kJ/min
Heavy	20.9 - 31.4 kJ/min
Very heavy	>31.4 kJ/min

*Based on the categorization of reference 14.

Occupational Work

In the past, energy expenditures required by occupational work and the associated demands of transportation (on foot or on a bicycle) accounted for a major fraction of the total daily metabolism in a large segment of the labor force (24). This is still true in some developing societies (17), and even in the western world occasional occupational categories with a high energy demand can still be distinguished.

Heavy occupational demand has had considerable epidemiological interest (56) in the past, because it has typically been sustained for 30-40 hours per week over many years. However, in modern post-industrial societies there now tends to be an inverted gradient between "heavy" employment and daily energy expenditure, since leisure activities that are differentially accessible to the wealthy constitute the main fraction of the total daily energy expenditure (15). The standards defining a high or a very high intensity of occupational activity (Table 2; 14) differ from those applicable to "exercise." This is because in industry the duration of individual activity bouts is usually prolonged, often there are other adverse circumstances (such as a high environmental temperature, an awkward posture, or a heavy loading of small muscle groups), and normally the pace of working is set by such factors as a machine, a supervisor, or a union contract, rather than the individual.

Household and Other Chores

Automation has progressively reduced the energy demands associated with the operation of a household in developed societies, largely outdating the figures cited in the classical literature (24). While some individuals may deliberately seek out heavy activities such as sawing logs, most necessary domestic chores now fall into the "light" category of the industrial scale. The one possible exception is the care of dependents. Both playing with young children and the nursing of elderly relatives can involve quite heavy work.

Dose-Response

As with administration of a drug, there appears to be a relationship between the dose of physical activity—its mode, frequency, intensity, and duration—and the biological response in terms of improvement of fitness and health. The dose-response relationship is characterized by (a) a threshold below which little or no adaptation occurs, (b) a zone of increasing effect, and (c) a ceiling beyond which no further improvement is observed or signs of over-dosage may develop. As age increases, the margin between an effective and an excessive quantity of exercise narrows, with a corresponding requirement for a more careful prescription of physical activity. However, the dose-response issue is quite complex and needs to be

considered in light of the diversity of the fitness components and health objectives.

The effects of a single dose of exercise may persist for several hours or days; thus, it is important to understand the interaction between the intensity, frequency, and duration of physical activity in determining the response.

Habitual Physical Activity

Physical activity is almost universally accepted as relevant to health, although the optimum pattern of activity (mode, intensity, frequency, and duration of individual bouts), interactions with nutritional status, and the cumulative impact of many years of participation, remain to be elucidated. It is desirable to combine the information on leisure physical activity, exercise, sports, occupational work, and other chores to assess the overall level of regular engagement in physical activity.

There is a need to integrate information on the intensity, frequency, and duration of physical activity to establish the pattern of activity over defined periods of time. One method of integration is to convert all data to an average weekly (leisure) energy expenditure (56). A second option is to compute an estimate of average 24-hour energy expenditure (28).

Energy Expenditure

The body conforms to the principle of the conservation of energy. Thus, long-term changes in an individual's body mass reflect the balance between their personal energy ingestion and energy expenditure. The liberation of heat energy by the body is expressed in joules, as an absolute value, as a ratio to estimated body surface area, per kilogram of body mass, or per kilogram of lean tissue mass. Important elements of overall daily energy expenditure in both sexes are the basal or resting metabolic rate, the energy cost of physical activity, and the thermic effect of food. In women, added demands are imposed by pregnancy and lactation.

In most circumstances, basal and resting metabolism account for the largest proportion of the individual's total daily energy expenditure. The rate of basal energy expenditure is relatively stable, although, if expressed per unit of body surface or body mass, it does show a small and progressive decrease with age. Small (about 10%) increases of resting metabolic rate are induced by ingesting a plethora of food (60), prolonged cold exposure (64), and possibly habitual activity or training (52);

whereas restriction of food intake tends to reduce basal and resting metabolic rate.

Physical activity is clearly the most variable component of the total daily energy expenditure. Depending on the fitness of the individual, a five- to twenty-fold increase of metabolic rate can be sustained for a few minutes, and a healthy young adult can, if necessary, develop five to eight times the basal metabolic rate over an 8 hour working day. In a very sedentary elderly person, the total daily energy usage can be as low as 6 MJ, whereas in a highly active ultra-long distance athlete, expenditures can reach 30 to 40 MJ.

Basal and resting metabolism, the increase of metabolism following a meal, and the sustained increase of metabolism following exercise can all be assessed under the carefully controlled experimental conditions of a metabolic ward. Doubly-labelled water has been used to determine CO_2 production and thus to infer total energy expenditure over periods of 1 to 2 weeks (44), although such observations are relatively costly. If food intake can be assessed accurately for several weeks, and if body mass remains constant, then there is a 10 to 15% concordance between the individual's intake and expenditure of energy.

Health-Related Fitness

In general terms, fitness can be conceived as the matching of the individual to his or her physical and social environment. However, there is no universally agreed upon definition of fitness and of its components. The World Health Organization (75) defined fitness as "the ability to perform muscular work satisfactorily." In keeping with this definition, fitness implies that the individual has attained those characteristics that permit a good performance of a given physical task in a specified physical, social, and psychological environment. The components of fitness are numerous and are determined by several variables including the individual's pattern and level of habitual activity, diet, and heredity.

Fitness is operationalized in present day Western societies with a focus on two goals: performance and health. Performance-related fitness refers to those components of fitness that are necessary for optimal work or sport performance (10,29,57,58). It is defined in terms of the individual's ability in athletic competition, a performance test, or occupational work. Performance-related fitness depends heavily upon motor skills, cardio-respiratory power and capacity, muscular strength, power or endurance, body size, body composition, motivation, and nutritional status. In general, performance-related fitness shows a limited relationship to health (57).

Health-related fitness refers to those components of fitness that are affected favorably or unfavorably by habitual physical activity and relate to health status. It has been defined as a state characterized by (a) an ability to perform daily activities with vigor and (b) demonstration of traits and capacities that are associated with a low risk of premature development of hypokinetic diseases and conditions (58). Important components of health-related fitness include body mass for height, body composition, subcutaneous fat distribution, abdominal visceral fat, bone density, strength and endurance of the abdominal and dorso-lumbar musculature, heart and lung function, blood pressure, maximal aerobic power and capacity, glucose and insulin metabolism, blood lipid and lipoprotein profile, and the ratio of lipid to carbohydrate oxidized in a variety of situations. A favorable profile for these various factors presents a clear advantage in terms of health outcomes as assessed by morbidity and mortality statistics.

Fitness is best understood in terms of the components that should be taken into consideration for its assessment, and the context in which the concept is operationalized. There are various ways of defining the components of fitness and we are proposing an approach which, we believe, takes into consideration the most recent achievements in exercise and clinical sciences (see Table 2.3). They include morphological, muscular, motor, cardiorespiratory, and metabolic fitness components.

Morphological Component

The morphological component of physical and physiological fitness can be defined in terms of several factors that are associated with various morbid conditions and mortality rate.

The *weight for height* (or the *body mass for height*) relationship is often expressed as the body mass index (body mass in kg divided by height in m²). High and very low body mass index values are both related to a higher all-cause mortality rate (72,73). Excessive weight for height is also associated with a greater likelihood of impaired glucose tolerance, hyperinsulinemia, hypertension, hypertriglyceridemia, and some dyslipoproteinemias (30,53,67). Body mass indices in the range of 20 to 25 are considered desirable among young adults

Table 2.3   The Components and Factors of Health-Related Fitness

Morphological component
  Body mass for height
  Body composition
  Subcutaneous fat distribution
  Abdominal visceral fat
  Bone density
  Flexibility

Muscular component
  Power
  Strength
  Endurance

Motor component
  Agility
  Balance
  Coordination
  Speed of movement

Cardiorespiratory component
  Submaximal exercise capacity
  Maximal aerobic power
  Heart functions
  Lung functions
  Blood pressure

Metabolic component
  Glucose tolerance
  Insulin sensitivity
  Lipid and lipoprotein metabolism
  Substrate oxidation characteristics

(35). Desirable values tend to shift slightly upward with age (body mass indices of 26 and 27; 2).

It is commonly accepted that *body fat content* is the source of the risk of morbidity and mortality associated with a high body mass index. However, there is no epidemiological study that has assessed the relationship between total body fat content and health outcomes. Nonetheless, small-scale laboratory studies indicate that percentage of body fat and fat mass are significantly correlated with blood lipid, lipoprotein, insulin levels, and blood pressure (19,45,50). In most cases, body composition has not been assessed by one of the direct methods but has been inferred from some combinations of body weight, body mass index, and skinfolds. The results of these studies are, however, consistent with those in which body composition was determined from underwater weighing or other well-accepted methods.

Subcutaneous fat distribution is considered as an important indicator of enhanced risk for cardiovascular disease morbidity and mortality and of

non-insulin dependent diabetes mellitus (8). A male profile of regional fat distribution (a preponderance of fat on the trunk) is associated with insulin resistance and elevated blood insulin level (25,38, 42), a more atherogenic plasma lipid and lipoprotein profile (18,41), and a higher blood pressure (19,38). A high proportion of fat over the upper-half of the body is also associated with a higher mortality rate in both sexes (46,47). Studies in which the amount of fat on the trunk has been assessed by skinfolds or by computerized tomography indicate that both the metabolic alterations and the increased cardiovascular mortality rates are associated with this profile of fat distribution (18,22,23,36).

In addition to the effects of an accumulation of trunco-abdominal subcutaneous fat on the risk profile, *abdominal visceral fat* also exerts a profound influence on insulin and lipoprotein metabolism (18,27,43). Within the abdominal visceral depot, it is thought that fat depots draining to the portal circulation are those that exert the largest adverse effects on hepatic glucose, lipid, and insulin metabolism (3). The amount of abdominal visceral fat can only be assessed by computerized tomography or other medical imaging techniques. In other words, it is useful to distinguish a minimum of three morphological factors and not only the total amount of body fat content but also the percent fat or fat mass, the trunco-abdominal subcutaneous fat, and the abdominal visceral fat (5). Lower body fat (the female pattern of fat deposition) apparently has only limited metabolic implications.

Bone mass is measured as local radiographic density or total body calcium. It is maximal in the third or fourth decade of life. There follows a progressive decrease of *bone density* which may progress to clinical osteoporosis and an increased susceptibility to bone fracture. Risk factors for osteoporosis include inherited susceptibility, a decrease in estrogen levels, a calcium deficient diet, and a low level of habitual physical activity (65). As osteoporosis reaches epidemic levels among the senior citizens of the developed countries of the western hemisphere, it is of great importance to understand the associations between habitual physical activity, fitness, and bone density. Currently available data support the notion that some types of physical activity may exert beneficial effects on bone mineral content and bone strength (54,65,69). In the context of bone health and overall skeletal strength, it is also useful to recognize that cartilage, ligaments, and tendons are favorably influenced by repeated muscular contractions (54,69).

Another factor of some importance in the morphological component of fitness is *flexibility*, generally defined as the range of motion at a joint. Flexibility is specific for a given joint and is determined by a variety of factors including the bony and cartilagenous surfaces and the soft tissues around the articulation. It can be improved by specific exercise designed to increase the range of motion at that particular joint. Although the issue is not yet entirely clear, it has been suggested that maintaining normal joint flexibility may help in preventing some of the manifestations of upper and lower back pain and osteoarthritis.

Muscular Component

Muscular fitness is universally recognized as an important component of physical and physiological fitness. Three factors are of particular interest: muscular power, muscular strength, and muscular endurance. *Muscular power* is strictly the maximum rate of working of a muscle, measured in a single effort such as a vertical jump. However, muscular power is sometimes taken as the peak power developed on an external device for as long as five seconds. *Muscular strength* can include the maximum force using an "isometric" dynamometer, an isokinetic dynamometer, or one repetition maximal isotonic lifting device. *Muscular endurance* is usually expressed as the decrease of peak force with a specified number of repetitions of an isokinetic or isotonic contraction. All three factors can be improved regardless of sex or age, given an appropriate regimen of exercise. Habitual activity does not appear to alter the slope of the aging curve, but the physically active person begins from a higher level of function and may thus experience less health impairment at a later age (63).

The progressive loss of lean tissue and muscular fitness with aging leads to a situation where desired activities such as lifting a load from the floor, carrying groceries, or lifting the body from a chair become impossible (63). Strong muscles also contribute to functional health by reducing the loading of joint surfaces, increasing the stability of articulations, and allowing a greater perfusion of the active fibers for any given absolute force of muscle contraction (16,39). A person with a reasonable level of muscular fitness should thus be less liable to local ischemia, with less fatigue, greater endurance, and a smaller rise in blood pressure as exercise continues.

It has been suggested that muscular fitness may be helpful in the prevention of upper and lower back pain that is so common in industrialized societies. Maintaining a reasonable level of muscular fitness through regular physical activity may also be important for normal hormonal and substrate metabolism, particularly for the insulin sensitivity of the active skeletal muscle tissue (26).

Motor Component

Motor fitness is of particular importance during growth, when the child explores his or her movement potential and develops basic motor skills. Agility, balance, speed of movement, and motor coordination are major facets of the motor component of fitness. *Agility* is usually described as a high score on a test that requires agile movements, such as a shuttle run. *Balance*, likewise, is described by scores on various tests of whole body equilibrium, or by measures of body sway. *Speed of movement* and *motor coordination* are characterized by fast responses to simple and complex choice reaction tasks. Motor fitness contributes only marginally to physical and physiological fitness as seen in a health perspective, with the possible exception of preventing falls and avoiding accidents, particularly in elderly people.

Cardiorespiratory Component

The cardiorespiratory component of physical and physiological fitness has traditionally been seen as the most important from a health point of view. Although this is still the case, important nuances are beginning to emerge (11). Cardiorespiratory fitness can be defined in terms of a large number of factors, the most relevant of which are listed in Table 3.

Submaximal exercise capacity or endurance performance can be defined as the tolerance to low intensity power output for prolonged periods of time. It is determined primarily by the oxygen delivery system, but is also affected by the peripheral utilization of oxygen to regenerate ATP, substrate mobilization and utilization, thermoregulatory mechanisms, and other physiological and metabolic factors. A person with a poor submaximal exercise capacity will experience fatigue sooner and may find problems in undertaking the normal activities of daily life.

Maximal aerobic power is assessed by measuring the maximal oxygen intake of the individual. Maximal oxygen intake decreases by about 10% per decade throughout adult life (63). The elderly individual becomes adversely affected by this decrease as some of the tasks of normal daily life require an increasingly large fraction of the maximal aerobic power. The initial maximal aerobic power is correlated with health outcomes (4), particularly with cardiovascular disease, and some (49) but not all authors (20,55) have also found an effect on non-insulin dependent diabetes mellitus risk factors.

Heart functions are assessed by a variety of indicators, including the cardiovascular response to exercise. The heart rate for a given power output (adjusted for body mass), the exercise stroke volume and cardiac output, the exercise electrocardiogram and vectocardiogram, and various imaging techniques that assess myocardium perfusion are among such indicators.

Lung functions may be assessed by measuring static and dynamic lung volumes. In most circumstances, the cardiorespiratory fitness of a healthy adult is limited by cardiac rather than by respiratory function. Nevertheless, it is ultimately better to have larger pulmonary volumes and higher flow rates for several reasons. One such reason is so a person can have a functional margin to accomodate the hazards of exposure to cigarette smoke, industrial dusts, other air pollutants, and respiratory pathogens.

Blood pressure is of particular importance, because hypertension is associated with an increased risk of death from ischemic heart disease, cardiac failure, cerebrovascular accident, rupture of other major blood vessels, and renal failure. There may also be some disadvantages to a very low systemic blood pressure, particularly a tendency to faint on standing suddenly after a period of recumbency. Regular physical activity and an improved fitness level may have positive influences on both hypotensive or hypertensive states (31,37). In addition to resting measurements of blood pressure, further information can be derived from the blood pressure response to exercise.

Metabolic Component

Metabolic fitness results from adequate hormonal actions, particularly for insulin, normal blood and tissue carbohydrate, and lipid metabolism. A high ratio of lipid to carbohydrate oxidized also seems to be a desirable trait.

Glucose tolerance is improved by regular physical activity; the response to training is generally better in those with an initially impaired glucose tolerance (26). Plasma insulin levels decrease (48,70) with hyperinsulinemic patients responding best to regular physical activity (26). Such changes are seen with programs of walking (48) and other low intensity, long duration, exercise sessions that do not necessarily cause an increase of maximal oxygen intake (12,55,70). It is not fully established whether the insulin-lowering effect of regular physical activity and the apparent improvement of an insulin-resistant state result from an acute or a short-term persistent increase in the *insulin sensitivity* of skeletal muscle and other peripheral tissues, because of a reduction in insulin secretion, an increased rate of hepatic removal of insulin, or a combination of these mechanisms.

Lipid metabolism is also an important dimension of metabolic fitness. Low plasma triglycerides, total cholesterol, low-density lipoprotein cholesterol, and high plasma high-density lipoprotein cholesterol are generally recognized as characteristics associated with a low risk of atherosclerotic diseases, particularly coronary heart disease. Regular physical activity is thought to alter lipid transport in the direction of this favorable profile (34,74). There are indications that the lipid profile may be favorably altered with exercise at a lower intensity than has generally been thought to be required (33,48,66,71).

Finally, *substrate oxidation characteristics* under standardized conditions at rest or during steady-state exercise are important indicators of metabolic efficiency. For instance, the respiratory quotient as measured over a 24-hour period in a metabolic chamber is significantly correlated with the amount of fat and weight gained over a period of about two years (76). Oxidizing more lipids than carbohydrates in a variety of conditions seems to be a desirable metabolic characteristic from a performance, fitness, and weight control point of view.

Health

Defining health remains a major challenge, despite the progress made in treating diseases and increasing the average life duration in Western societies. At the 1988 Consensus Conference (10), health was defined as a human condition with physical, social, and psychological dimensions, each characterized on a continuum with positive and negative poles. Positive health is associated with a capacity to enjoy life and to withstand challenges; it is not merely the absence of disease. Negative health is associated with morbidity and, in the extreme, with premature mortality.

Morbidity can be defined as any departure, subjective or objective, from a state of physical or psychological well-being, short of death. Morbidity is measured as (a) the number of persons who are ill per unit of population per year, (b) the incidence of specific conditions per unit of population per year, and (c) the average duration of these conditions. On the other hand, wellness is a holistic concept, describing a state of positive health in the individual, and comprising physical, social, and psychological well-being.

Traditional illness and mortality statistics do not provide a full assessment of health as conceived in the context of this paper. A more comprehensive approach would require that the risk profile of the individual be established in terms of common health endpoints, an assessment of health-related fitness status, information on temporary and chronic disabilities, absenteeism, overall productivity, and use of all forms of medical services, including prescribed and non-prescribed drugs. If the quality of life is less than optimal, life expectancy should be adjusted to reflect a quality-adjusted value. This reflects the individual's summated quality of life on each of a range of criteria at each point in their lifespan.

Other Factors Affecting Physical Activity, Fitness, and Health

Three types of influence are important: lifestyle factors other than physical activity level, physical environment, and social environment and personal attributes.

Lifestyle

Lifestyle comprises the aggregate of an individual's actions and behaviors of choice which can affect health-related fitness and health status. Habitual physical activity is one such behavior over which the individual has a large measure of voluntary control. In addition, we are particularly concerned by smoking, diet (energy intake and dietary composition), and alcohol consumption as they impact health-related fitness and health in general. The association between habitual physical activity and other favorable lifestyle behaviors is in the expected direction but is not very strong. However, the relationship is strengthened if emphasis is placed upon those facets of physical activity that are undertaken with the deliberate intention of promoting health.

An understanding of the role of lifestyle on fitness and health should also include an assessment of sleeping patterns, perceived stress, drug addiction, and the general avoidance of health risks, such as wearing a seat belt; observing traffic regulations; scheduling regular medical, dental, and self-examinations; and avoiding hazardous sexual behavior (13,15).

Social Environment and Personal Attributes

In the present context, the social environment may be defined as the combination of social, cultural, political, and economic conditions that affect participation in physical activity, health-related fitness, and health status. Social networks may have a positive influence on attitudes toward physical activity and other healthy behaviors. Friends, members of the family, other relatives, social clubs, church organizations, and other groups are all part of the social milieu that can affect both health and the sense of well-being of an individual. All these elements of the social network can provide support for active living, but can also exert powerful influences in the opposite direction. Thus, a healthy public policy strives to provide political, economic, and cultural conditions conducive to good health practices. Examples are encouragement of bicycle commuting, restrictions on smoking in public places, and a building design that encourages stair climbing.

Several personal attributes shape the lifestyle pattern of a person, including the attitude toward physical activity and other healthy habits. These attributes include age, gender, socioeconomic status, personality characteristics, and motivation.

Physical Environment

Participation in leisure time physical activity, fitness level, and health status are all influenced by environmental conditions. These include temperature, humidity, air quality, altitude and climatic changes. Such conditions influence not only the ability to exercise, but also the physiological response to the demands of exercise. Certain types of physical activity may be hazardous to health because of prevailing environmental conditions.

Heredity and Individual Differences

Health is the culmination of many interacting factors, including the genetic constitution. The genotype represents the characteristics of the individual at a given gene or set of genes. Humans are genetically quite diverse; current estimates are that each human being has about one variable DNA base for every 100 to 300 bases. Variations in DNA sequence constitute the molecular basis of genetic individuality and of human genetic variation. Given these circumstances, an equal state of health and of physical and mental well-being is unlikely to be achieved for all. Some will thrive better and will remain free from disabilities for a longer period of time than others.

Genetic differences do not operate in a vacuum. They interact constantly with existing cellular and tissue conditions to provide a biological response commensurate with environmental demands. In that sense, the genes are constantly interacting with everything in the physical and social environment, as well as with lifestyle characteristics of the individual, that translate into a signal capable of affecting the cells of the body. Thus, overfeeding, a high fat diet, smoking, and regular endurance exercise are all powerful stimuli that may elicit strong biological responses. However, because of inherited differences at specific genes, the amplitude of adaptive responses varies from one individual to the other. Inheritance is one of the important reasons why we are not equally prone to diabetes, hypertension, or heart attacks. It is also one major explanation for individual differences in the response to dietary intervention or exercise training.

Genetic individuality is important in the present context because it has an impact on the physical activity, fitness, and health paradigm. Thus, there are inherited differences in the level of habitual physical activity (59) and for many components of health-related fitness (6,9). There is now highly suggestive evidence that genetic variation accounts for a substantial fraction of the individual differences in the response to regular exercise of health-related fitness factors and the various risk factors for cardiovascular disease and non-insulin dependent diabetes mellitus (7,9,10).

A recognition of the critical role of DNA sequence variation in human response to a variety of challenges and environmental conditions seems essential to all those interested in the physical activity, fitness, and health paradigm. It will augment our understanding of human variation and make us more cautious in defining fitness and health benefits that may be anticipated from a physically active lifestyle. Incorporating biological individuality into our thinking can only increase the relevance of our observations to the true human situation.

References

1. American College of Sports Medicine. The recommended quantity and quality of exercise for developing and maintaining cardiorespiratory and muscular fitness in healthy adults. *Med. Sci. Sports Exerc.* 22: 265-274; 1990.

2. Andres, R. Mortality and Obesity: The rationale for age-specific height-weight tables. In: Andres, R.; Bierman, E.L.; Hazzard, W.R. eds. *Principles of geriatric medicine.* New York: McGraw-Hill; 1985: 311-318.

3. Björntorp, P. Portal adipose tissue as a generator of risk factors for cardiovascular disease and diabetes. *Arteriosclerosis.* 10: 493-496; 1990.

4. Blair, S.N.; Kohl, H.W. III; Paffenbarger, R.S. Jr.; Clark, D.G.; Cooper, K.H.; Gibbons, L.W. Physical fitness and all-causes mortality: A prospective study of healthy men and women. *JAMA* 262: 2395-2401; 1989.

5. Bouchard, C. Heredity and the path to overweight and obesity. *Med. Sci. Sports Exerc.* 23: 285-291; 1991.

6. Bouchard, C. Genetic determinants of endurance performance. In: Shephard, R.J., Astrand, P.O. eds. *Endurance in sports.* Oxford: Blackwell Scientific, Vol. II of the Encyclopedia of Sports Medicine an IOC Medical Commission Publication; 1992: 149-159.

7. Bouchard, C. Discussion: Heredity, fitness, and health. In: Bouchard, C.; Shephard, R.J.; Stephens, T.; Sutton, J.R.; McPherson, B.D.; eds. *Exercise, fitness and health: A consensus of current knowledge.* Champaign, IL: Human Kinetics; 1990: 147-153.

8. Bouchard, C.; Bray, G.A.; Van Hubbard, V.S. Basic and clinical aspects of regional fat distribution. *Am. J. Clin. Nutr.* 52: 946-950; 1990.

9. Bouchard, C.; Dionne, F.T.; Simoneau, J.A.; Boulay, M.R. Genetics of aerobic and anaerobic performances. *Exerc. Sport Sci. Rev.* 1992, 20: 27-58.

10. Bouchard, C.; Shephard, R.J.; Stephens, T.; Sutton, J.R.; McPherson, B.D. *Exercise, fitness and health: a consensus of current knowledge.* Champaign, IL: Human Kinetics; 1990.

11. Bouchard, C.; Shephard, R.J.; Stephens, T.; Sutton, J.R.; McPherson, B.D. Exercise, fitness and health: the consensus statement. In: Bouchard, C.; Shephard, R.J.; Stephens, T.; Sutton, J.R.; McPherson, B.D.; eds. *Exercise, fitness and health: a consensus of current knowledge.* Champaign, IL: Human Kinetics; 1990: 3-28.

12. Bouchard, C.; Tremblay, A.; Nadeau, A.; Dussault, J.; Després, J.P.; Thériault, G.; Lupien, P.J.; Serresse, O.; Boulay, M.R.; Fournier, G. Long-term exercise training with constant energy intake. 1: Effect on body composition and selected metabolic variables. *Int. J. Obes.* 14: 57-73; 1990.

13. Breslow, L. Lifestyle, fitness, and health. In: Bouchard, C.; Shephard, R.J.; Stephens, T.; Sutton, J.R.; McPherson, B.D.; eds. *Exercise, fitness and health: A consensus of current knowledge.* Champaign, IL: Human Kinetics; 1990: 155-163.

14. Brown, J.R.; Crowden, G.P. Energy expenditure ranges and muscular work grades. *Br. J. Industr. Med.* 20: 277-283; 1963.

15. Canada Fitness Survey. *Fitness and lifestyle in Canada.* Ottawa: Directorate of fitness and amateur sport; 1983.

16. Clausen, J.P. Muscle blood flow during exercise and its significance for maximal performance. In: Keul, J.; ed. *Limiting factors of physical performance.* Stuttgart: Thieme Verlag; 1973: 253-266.

17. Collins, K. Energy expenditure, productivity and endemic disease. In: Harrison, G.A., ed. *Energy and effort.* London: Taylor and Francis; 1982: 65-84.

18. Després, J.P.; Moorjani, S.; Lupien, P.J.; Tremblay, A.; Nadeau, A.; Bouchard, C. Regional fat distribution of body fat, plasma lipoproteins, and cardiovascular disease. *Arteriosclerosis* 10: 497-511; 1990.

19. Després, J.P.; Tremblay, A.; Thériault, G.; Pérusse, L.; Leblanc, C.; Bouchard, C. Relationships between body fatness, adipose tissue distribution, and blood pressure in men and women. *J. Clin. Epidemiol.* 41: 889-897; 1988.

20. Després, J.P.; Moorjani, S.; Tremblay, A.; Poehlman, E.T.; Lupien, P.J.; Nadeau, A.; Bouchard, C. Heredity and changes in plasma lipids and lipoproteins after short-term exercise training in men. *Arteriosclerosis.* 8: 402-409; 1988.

21. Dishman, R.K. Determinants of participation in physical activity. In: Bouchard, C.; Shephard, R.J.; Stephens, T.; Sutton, J.R.; McPherson, B.D.; eds. *Exercise, fitness and health: a consensus of current knowledge.* Champaign, IL: Human Kinetics; 1990: 75-101.

22. Ducimetière, P.; Richard, J.L. The relationship between subsets of anthropometric upper versus lower body measurements and coronary heart disease risk in middle-aged men. The Paris prospective study. *Int. J. Obes.* 13: 111-112; 1989.

23. Ducimetière, P.; Richard, J.L.; Cambien, F. The pattern of subcutaneous fat distribution in middle-aged men and the risk of coronary heart disease. The Paris prospective study. *Int. J. Obes.* 10: 229-240; 1986.

24. Durnin, J.V.G.A; Passmore, R. *Energy, work and leisure.* London: Heinemann; 1967.

25. Evans, D.J.; Hoffman R.G.; Kalkhoff, R.K. Kissebah, A.H. Relationship of body fat topography to insulin sensitivity and metabolic profiles in premenopausal women. *Metabolism.* 33: 68-75; 1984.

26. Exercise and NIDDM. *Diabetes Care.* 13: 785-789; 1990.

27. Fujioka, S.; Matsuzawa, Y.; Tokunaga, K.; Tarui, S. Contribution of intra-abdominal fat accumulation to the impairment of glucose and lipid metabolism in human obesity. *Metabolism.* 36: 54-59; 1987.

28. Furrie, A.D.; Stephens, T. Energy expenditure patterns in the Canadian population. In: Landry, F., ed. *Health risk estimation, risk reduction and health promotion.* Ottawa: Canadian Public Health Association; 1983: 103-114.

29. Gledhill, N. Discussion: Assessment of Fitness. In: Bouchard, C.; Shephard, R.J.; Stephens, T.; Sutton, J.R.; McPherson, B.D.; eds. *Exercise, fitness and health: a consensus of current knowledge.* Champaign, IL: Human Kinetics; 1990.

30. Glueck, C.J.; Taylor, H.L.; Jacobs, D.; Morrisson, J.A.; Beaglehole, R.; Williams, O.D. Plasma high-density lipoprotein cholesterol: Association with measurements of body mass. *The Lipid Research Clinics Prevalence Study.* Circulation 62 (suppl IV): 62-69; 1980.

31. Hagberg, J.M. Exercise, fitness, and hypertension. In: Bouchard, C.; Shephard, R.J.; Stephens, T.; Sutton, J.R.; McPherson, B.D.; eds. *Exercise, fitness and health: A consensus of current knowledge.* Champaign, IL: Human Kinetics; 1990: 455-466.

32. Hanke, H. *Freizeit in der DDR.* Berlin: Dietz Verlag; 1979.

33. Hardman, A.E.; Hudson, A.; Jones, P.R.M.; Norgan, N.G. Brisk walking and plasma high density lipoprotein cholesterol concentration in previously sedentary women. *Br. Med. J.* 299: 1204-1205; 1989.

34. Haskell, W.L. The influence of exercise training on plasma lipids and lipoproteins in health and disease. *Acta. Med. Scand.* Suppl 711: 25-37; 1986.

35. Health and Welfare Canada. Canadian guidelines for healthy weights. Ottawa: Supplies and Services Canada; 1989.

36. Higgins, M.; Kannel, W.; Garrison, R.; Pinsky, J.; Stokes, J. Hazards of obesity—The Framingham experience. *Acta. Med. Scand. Suppl.* 723: 23-36; 1988.

37. Holmgren, A. Vaso-regulatory asthenia. *Can. Med. Assoc. J.* 96: 853; 1967.

38. Kalkhoff, R.K.; Hartz, A.H.; Rupley, D.; Kissebah, A.H.; Kelber, S. Relationship of body fat distribution to blood pressure, carbohydrate tolerance, and plasma lipids in healthy obese women. *J. Lab. Clin. Med.* 102: 621-627; 1983.

39. Kay, C.; Shephard, R.J. On muscle strength and the threshold of anaerobic work. *Int. Z. Angew. Physiol.* 27: 311-328; 1969.

40. Kenyon, G.S. Six scales for assessing attitudes towards physical activity. *Res. Quart.* 39: 566-574; 1968.

41. Kissebah, A.H.; Vydelingum, N.; Murray, R.; Evans, D.V.; Hartz, A.J.; Kalkhoff, R.K.; Adams, P.W. Relation of body fat distribution to metabolic complications of obesity. *J. Clin. Endocrinol. Metab.* 54: 254-260; 1982.

42. Kissebah, A.H.; Peiris, A.N. Biology of regional body fat distribution: Relationship to non-insulin dependent diabetes mellitus. *Diabetes Metab. Rev.* 5: 83-109; 1989.

43. Kissebah, A.H.; Freedman, D.S.; Peiris, A.N. Health risks of obesity. *Med. Clin. North Am.* 73: 111-138; 1989.

44. Klein, P.D.; James, W.P.; Wong, W.W.; Irving, C.S.; Murgatroyd, P.R.; Cabrera, M. Dalosso, H.M.; Klein, E.R.; Nichols, B.L. Calorimetric validation of the doubly labeled water method for estimation of energy expenditure in man. *Hum. Nutr. Clin. Nutr.* 38: 95-106; 1984.

45. Krotkiewski, M.; Björntorp, P.; Sjöstrom, L.; Smith, U. Impact of obesity on metabolism in men and women. Importance of regional adipose tissue distribution. *J. Clin. Invest.* 72: 1150-1162; 1983.

46. Lapidus, L.; Benftsson, C.; Larsson, B.; Pennert, K.; Rybo, E.; Sjöström, L. Distribution of adipose tissue and risk of cardiovascular disease and death: A 12-year follow-up of participants in the population study of women in Gothenburg, Sweden. *Br. Med. J.* 289: 1261-1263; 1984.

47. Larsson, B.; Svardsudd K.; Welin, L.; Wilhelmsen, L.; Björntorp, P.; Tibblin, G. Abdominal adipose tissue distribution, obesity and risk of cardiovascular disease and death 13 year follow-up of participants in the study of men born in 1913. *Br. Med. J.* 288: 1401-1404; 1984.

48. Leon, A.S.; Conrad, J.; Hunninghake, D.B.; Serfass, R. Effects of a vigorous walking program on body composition, carbohydrate and lipid metabolism of obese young men. *Am. J. Clin. Nutr.* 32: 1776-1787; 1979.

49. Leon, A.S.; Connett, J.; Jacobs, D.R. Jr.; Rauramaa, R. Leisure time physical activity levels and risk of heart disease and death: The Multiple Risk Factor Intervention Trial. *JAMA,* 258: 2388-2395; 1987.

50. Mauriège, P.; Després, J.P.; Marcotte, M.; Ferland, M.; Tremblay, A.; Nadeau, A.; Moorjani, S.; Lupien, P.J.; Thériault, G.; Bouchard, C. Abdominal fat cell lipolysis, body fat distribution, and metabolic variables in premenopausal women. *J. Clin. Endocrinol. Metab.* 71: 1028-1035; 1990.

51. McIntosh, P.C. *"Sport for All" programmes throughout the world.* Paris: UNESCO contract 207604; 1980.

52. Molé, P. Impact of energy intake and exercise on resting metabolic rate. *Sports Med.* 10: 72-87; 1990.

53. National Research Council. *Diet and health. Implications for reducing chronic disease risk.* Washington, DC: National Academy Press: 1989: 563-592.

54. Oakes, B.W.; Parker, A.W. Discussion: Bone and connective tissue adaptations to physical activity. In: Bouchard, C.; Shephard, R.J.; Stephens, T.; Sutton, J.R.; McPherson, B.D.; eds. *Exercise, fitness and health: a consensus of current knowledge.* Champaign, IL: Human Kinetics; 1990: 345-361.

55. Oshida, Y.; Yamanonchi, K.; Hazamizu, S.; Sato, Y. Long-term mild jogging increases insulin action despite no influence on body mass index or $\dot{V}O_2$max. *J. Appl. Physiol.* 66: 2206-2210; 1989.

56. Paffenbarger, R.; Hyde, R.T.; Wing, A.L. Physical activity and physical fitness as determinants of health and longevity. In: Bouchard, C.; Shephard, R.J.; Stephens, T.; Sutton, J.R.; McPherson, B.D.; eds. *Exercise, fitness and health: a consensus of current knowledge.* Champaign, IL: Human Kinetics; 1990: 33-48.

57. Pate, R.R.; Shephard, R.J. Characteristics of physical fitness in youth. In: Gisolfi, C.V.; Lamb, D.R., eds. *Perspectives in exercise science and sports medicine, vol 2, Youth, exercise and sport.* Indianapolis, IN: Benchmark Press; 1989: 1-45.

58. Pate, R.R. The evolving definition of fitness. *Quest.* 40: 174-179; 1988.

59. Pérusse, L.; Tremblay, A.; Leblanc, C.; Bouchard, C. Genetic and familial environmental influences on level of habitual physical activity. *Am. J. Epidemiol.* 129: 1012-1022; 1989.

60. Rothwell, N.J.; Stocks, M.J. Luxuskonsumption, diet-induced thermogenesis—the case in favour. *Clin. Sci.* 64: 19-23; 1983.

61. Sachs, M.L. Compliance and addiction to exercise. In: Cantu RC, ed. *The exercising adult*. Lexington, MA: DA Heath; 1982: 19-27.

62. Shephard, R.J. *Endurance fitness (2nd ed)*. Toronto: University of Toronto Press; 1977.

63. Shephard, R.J. *Physical activity and aging (2nd ed)*. London: Croom Holm; 1987.

64. Shephard, R.J. Adaptation to exercise in the cold. *Sports Med.* 2: 59-71; 1985.

65. Smith, E.L.; Smith, K.A.; Gilligan, C. Exercise, fitness, osteoarthritis, and osteoporosis. In: Bouchard, C.; Shephard, R.J.; Stephens, T.; Sutton, J.R.; McPherson, B.D.; eds. *Exercise, fitness and health: a consensus of current knowledge*. Champaign, IL: Human Kinetics; 1990: 517-528.

66. Sopko, G.; Jacobs, D.R.; Jeffery, R.; Mittelmark, M.; Lenz, K.; Hedding, E.; Lipcjik, R.; Gerber, W. Effects on blood lipids and body weight in high risk men of a practical exercise program. *Atherosclerosis.* 49; 219-229; 1983.

67. Stamler, J. Overweight, hypertension, hypercholesterolemia and coronary heart disease. In: Mancini, M.; Lewis, B.; Contaldo, F., eds. *Medical complications of obesity*. London: Academic Press; 1979: 191-216.

68. Stundl, H. *Freizeit und Erholungsport in der DDR*. Schorndorf: Karl Hofmann Verlag; 1977.

69. Tipton, C.M.; Vailas, A.C. Bone and connective tissue adaptations to physical activity. In: Bouchard, C.; Shephard, R.J.; Stephens, T.; Sutton, J.R.; McPherson, B.D.; eds. *Exercise, fitness and health: a consensus of current knowledge*. Champaign, IL: Human Kinetics; 1990: 331-344.

70. Tremblay, A.; Nadeau, A.; Després, J.P.; St-Jean, L.; Thériault, G.; Bouchard, C. Long-term exercise training with constant energy intake. 2: Effect on glucose metabolism and resting energy expenditure. *Int. J. Obes.* 14: 75-84; 1990.

71. Tucker, L.A.; Friedman, G.M. Walking and serum cholesterol in adults. *Am. J. Publ. Health.* 80: 1111-1113; 1990.

72. Van Itallie, T.B.; Abraham, S. Some hazards of obesity and its treatment. In: Hirsch, J.; Van Itallie, T.B., eds. *Recent advances in obesity research IV*. London: John Libbey; 1985: 1-19.

73. Waaler, H. Height, weight and mortality. The Norwegian experience. *Acta. Med. Scand.,* Suppl 679; 1983.

74. Wood, P.D.; Stefanick, M.L. Exercise, fitness, and atherosclerosis. In: Bouchard, C.; Shephard, R.J.; Stephens, T.; Sutton, J.R.; McPherson, B.D.; eds. *Exercise, fitness and health: a consensus of current knowledge*. Champaign, IL: Human Kinetics; 1990: 409-423.

75. World Health Organization. Meeting of investigators on exercise tests in relation to cardiovascular function. *WHO Technical Report.* 388; 1968.

76. Zurlo, F.; Lilioja, S.; Esposito-Del Puente, A.; Nyomba, B.; Raz, I.; Saad, M.; Swinburn, B.; Knowler, W.; Bogardus, C.; Ravussin, E. Low ratio of fat to carbohydrate oxidation as predictor of weight gain. *Am. J. Physiol.* 259: E650-E657; 1990.

Chapter 3

Assessing the Level
and Quality of Evidence

A meaningful consensus document should provide clinicians and researchers with guidance based on current scientific evidence, rather than merely outlining recommendations supported by available literature. Although it is plausible to assert that only the conclusions derived from methodologically defensible studies should be included in consensus documents, the reality of the scientific process demands otherwise. In many instances, consensus guidelines have to draw on somewhat imperfect or incomplete evidence. Defining minimally acceptable criteria for the validity and applicability of published data is therefore essential. To assist with this sort of endeavor, clinical methodologists have developed a comprehensive set of critical appraisal criteria that can be used to scrutinize both clinical and basic science literature.

Criteria have been generated to evaluate studies that deal with clinical measurement, diagnosis, the effectiveness of treatment, prognosis, disease, causation, quality of care, and health economics. Study designs are carefully weighted within each of these categories. Overviews (either meta-analyses or traditional review articles) can also be appraised according to defined criteria. Although randomized control trials are usually considered the benchmark of robust methodology, the findings from studies with other designs merit consideration in instances where randomized control trials are either inappropriate or unavailable.

One study that examined the choice of research methodology in various areas of the sports sciences demonstrated that cohort and cross-sectional designs were the most popular choices, accounting for 72% of all epidemiological studies published in an arbitrary sample of the sports science literature over a 12 month period. A case series approach was identified in 13% of the papers and case control studies constituted 7% of the total. Only 8% of the published papers were randomized control trials.

When applying critical appraisal criteria to this body of literature, the author of this particular review suggested that randomization had not been used, when perhaps it should have been, in approximately six out of every seven therapeutic studies and in two of every three studies on sports physiology or biomechanics. Furthermore, many of the sample sizes reported in the survey would have given inadequate statistical power to support the hypotheses that were advanced. A tendency to overlook the inherent limitations of numerator-based data was a further perceived inadequacy in the spectrum of 756 papers included in the review.

These findings suggest that a higher standard of sports science research will be possible once investigators appreciate the potential advantages of stronger research designs and receive the level of funding required for larger and more sophisticated investigations.

Chapter 4

Assessment of Physical Activity, Fitness, and Health

Methods of Assessing Physical Activity During Leisure and Work

The various methods currently available to assess physical activity vary greatly in their applicability in epidemiologic research, intervention studies, clinical practice, and personal assessment. Many measurement problems stem from the fact that physical activity is a complex behavior which generally accounts for 15% to 40% of a person's total energy expenditure. This behavior encompasses physical activity on the job, self-care, household chores, home and yard maintenance, transportation, and discretionary leisure-time activities including fitness-promoting exercise and sports. Health-related dimensions include not only the contribution of physical activity to total energy expenditure, but intensity, duration, and frequency.

About 50 different individual assessment techniques are included under six general categories of physical activity assessment tools (see Table 4.1). Factors affecting selection of an appropriate measurement technique include: the nature of the problem under study; the dimension of physical activity related to health outcomes; the size and demographics of the study population; practicality in terms of cost; time to administer and process the measurements; appropriateness and acceptability to study subjects; compatibility and nonreactivity with usual daily activities; and the reliability and validity of the instrument used.

Calorimetry and doubly labeled water can provide accurate measurements of average daily energy expenditure under controlled laboratory conditions. The precise measurement of energy intake under conditions of weight maintenance also provides a good estimate of daily energy expenditure. In addition, behavioral observation techniques and physical activity diaries or records yield information about specific activity patterns. Although these methods are not practical for use in large population studies, they are useful with small samples and for validation of physical activity survey questionnaires. Other less accurate validation techniques commonly employed for validating survey instruments include heart rate monitoring, electronic and mechanical motion detection, and various measurements of physical fitness, particularly $\dot{V}O_2max$, and associations with chronic diseases (e.g., coronary heart disease).

Questionnaire methods are currently the most popular and practical approaches for large population studies because of the volume and detail of information that they provide relative to cost and time invested. Assignment of levels of physical activity according to specific job categories or occupational titles also has been commonly employed in population studies because of its simplicity; however, the accuracy of this technique for physical activity classification is questionable. Global self-reports, which require individuals to respond

Table 4.1 Physical Activity Assessment Procedures

1. Calorimetry:
   a) Direct heat exchange (in insulated chamber or "space-suit")
   b) Indirect (respirometry)

2. Physiologic markers:
   a) Heart rate monitoring
   b) Doubly isotopically labeled water
   c) Cardiorespiratory endurance ($\dot{V}O_2max$)

3. Mechanical and electronic motion detectors:
   a) Pedometer
   b) In-shoe step counters
   c) Electronic motion sensors
   d) Accelerometers

4. Behavioral observations

5. Dietary energy intake (food diary)

6. Occupational and leisure-time survey instruments:
   a) Job classification
   b) Global self-assessment
   c) Activity diaries or records
   d) Recall questionnaires
   e) Quantitative histories

to a limited number of simple questions about their usual physical activity habits, have good repeatability and fair validity. A wide variety of self- or interviewer-administered physical activity questionnaires of various lengths and complexities are currently available.

It is possible to select and/or score questionnaires to assess different physical activity dimensions. The length of the recall periods in these questionnaires generally varies from one week to a year, but some assess "usual" physical activity participation patterns, and the emphasis usually is on high intensity activities. The retrospective quantitative history (for example, the Minnesota Leisure-Time Physical Activity Questionnaire) is a more comprehensive form of survey procedure; it asks for the month-by-month frequency and duration of an extensive list of activities. The trade-off is greater cost, because increased time is required for administration and data processing.

IMPORTANT RESEARCH TOPICS

1. Standardized physical activity questionnaires are needed to identify and monitor secular trends over the entire spectrum of energy expenditure and dimensions of physical activity for representative samples of various populations and cultures in different areas of the world, including relevant subsets based on age and gender. Such questionnaires also can be useful for behavioral research to better define determinants of physical activity and exercise, and assess the effects of interventions.
2. The reliability and validity of existing and new physical activity questionnaires should be determined using existing and improved criteria standards.
3. Additional research is required to develop objective measures of physical activity (such as improved motion sensors) better suited to epidemiologic investigations, as well as for assessing clinical interventions and personal activity guidance.
4. There is a need to identify the most concise survey questions that reflect specific health-related dimensions of physical activity.
5. Basic research is also needed on how people encode, store, and recall specific information about physical activity.

Laboratory and Field Tests for Assessing Health-Related Fitness

In the assessment of physical and physiological fitness, it is important to identify whether the information relates to performance or health-related fitness. Most of the current methods for assessing fitness have evolved in the context of performance-related fitness. Their usefulness as measures of health-related fitness has not been systematically evaluated. It is important to distinguish between *performance-related norms* (e.g., below average, average, and above average) which are used to classify people in relation to their peers and *health-related criterion standards* (e.g., undesirable, minimal, acceptable, and desirable) which are used for screening, guidance, and encouragement. Most adults do not need to be tested. Instead, they need information about minimal and desirable levels of the various aspects of health-related fitness required for good health and independence. And they need to know about the amount and types of exercise needed to reach these levels. Unfortunately, little is known about the minimal levels of such factors as muscular strength or flexibility that are needed at different age groups and in different health states.

Morphological Fitness

For large scale practical assessment of body composition factors involved in health-related fitness, the body mass index, selected skinfolds from the limbs and trunk, and the waist to hip circumference ratio will provide reasonable estimates of (a) body fat content and (b) regional fat distribution (especially subcutaneous fat).

IMPORTANT RESEARCH TOPICS

6. More direct methods are needed to determine body composition. Simpler and more accurate indirect methods are also needed for field surveys. Further study is needed of the influence of such factors as age, gender, and disease upon population differences of body composition.
7. There is a need to modify techniques for the assessment of body composition, developing prediction equations and reference values that will allow the indirect assessment of body fatness, including regional fat distribution and the amount of abdominal visceral fat.

Bone Strength

In the context of health, bone strength is essentially synonymous with bone mineral density. The loss in bone mineral density with age is associated with a higher risk of osteoporosis and bone fractures. Exercise may lower the risk of fractures and osteoporosis by countering bone loss, by enhancing neuromuscular abilities that help to avert falls, and by reducing the impact if a fall occurs. Although there is evidence that exercise increases peak bone mass and attenuates the bone loss with age, the exact dose-response relationship between exercise and bone mineral density is not known. Densitometry is the best method to obtain useful, accurate information on bone mineral density, but will probably remain a research tool for some time to come. There are non-invasive methods to measure bone "stiffness," but too few studies have been carried out to evaluate their usefulness adequately.

IMPORTANT RESEARCH TOPICS

8. Simpler, inexpensive methods are needed to assess bone health.
9. Long-term prospective studies are needed to determine: (a) the health importance of bone "stiffness," (b) the sensitivity of densitometry and other indirect methods to measure the changes in bone mineral density and in bone stiffness that occur as a result of age or various interventions, and (c) the accuracy with which densitometric and other indirect methods can predict the risk of fractures in various populations.

Muscular Fitness

Although it is clear that strength and health are related, once strength falls below levels needed to accomplish the activities of daily living, the association among health, strength, and endurance of muscle groups other than the legs (e.g., those in the upper body) is poorly known. Research on health-related muscular fitness has focused on the possible role of a lack of trunk muscle strength and endurance in the development of back, neck, and shoulder problems. It is unclear what types and combinations of muscular fitness (isometric, isotonic, isokinetic power, strength, or endurance) are most important in this regard. The performance of specific muscle groups can be assessed in the laboratory, but this generally requires equipment be used under strictly controlled and standardized conditions. The practical health application of the data obtained remains questionable.

Traditional field tests of trunk-muscle fitness include repeat sit-ups and a variety of static or dynamic back extension tests. None of these procedures is fully satisfactory with respect to feasibility, safety, reliability, and validity when assessing large groups of individuals.

Flexibility

General flexibility is believed to be important for health, especially in terms of extending the period of independence in older adults. Trunk flexibility may also have health implications for back, neck, and shoulder problems. Several observational, cross-sectional studies have found that poor thoraco-lumbar and/or lumbar mobility may be related to an increased risk of back problems.

The static range of motion of specific joints can be assessed accurately in the laboratory, but there are problems of standardization and of equipment. Field assessment of trunk flexibility includes variations of the sit-and-reach and stand-and-reach tests. Maximal reach tests are affected by the relative length of upper and lower limbs, involve a significant tolerance component, and may be unsafe for some people. Interpretation of the results is difficult. Lateral spine bending is an unambiguous, simple, and safe test, but its health-related role is unknown.

IMPORTANT RESEARCH TOPICS

10. More studies are needed to establish firmly the relationship between musculoskeletal fitness and physical function or other aspects of health.
11. Criterion standards of trunk muscle strength and endurance and trunk mobility are needed in different populations, especially in older adults.
12. Standardized, feasible and safe field tests of muscle strength and endurance and flexibility are needed.
13. The validity, feasibility, safety and subject acceptability of most field tests of musculoskeletal fitness need to be studied in different populations.

Motor Fitness

Postural control can affect musculoskeletal health by decreasing the risk of falls which may lead to bone fractures. The assessment of postural control is a complex task and its complete determination may require several approaches using kinematic and biomechanical methods.

IMPORTANT RESEARCH TOPICS

14. More research is needed to establish the relationship between postural control and physical function as well as other aspects of health.
15. The scientific quality (validity, reliability, and feasibility) of the present tests of postural control needs to be assessed and new tests developed.

Cardiorespiratory Fitness

The two health-related components of cardiorespiratory fitness are maximal aerobic power and the ability to perform prolonged submaximal exercise (submaximal cardiorespiratory capacity). The traditional objective laboratory assessment of $\dot{V}O_2max$ usually requires a treadmill or a cycle ergometer, apparatus involving rhythmic, dynamic exercise with a large and standardized muscle mass capable of maximally stressing the systems for transporting and utilizing oxygen. For direct measurement of oxygen consumption, gas analysis equipment is needed.

It has been argued that cardiorespiratory capacity or efficiency during submaximal work may be important for reducing fatigue in heavy industry or, in an older person, extending the ability to undertake the activities of daily living. However, there is no direct evidence that the ability to perform prolonged submaximal exercise is related to health. While $\dot{V}O_2max$ is conceptually and methodologically unambiguous, the exact characteristics of submaximal cardiorespiratory capacity need to be defined, and appropriate assessment methods need to be developed. Measures of cardiovascular function during submaximal exercise may be useful in this regard.

There is little inherent reason to measure $\dot{V}O_2max$ for health-related purposes. If a submaximal procedure of adequate precision was available, a better approach might be to estimate maximal aerobic power from submaximal tests, so that large numbers of middle-aged and older adults could be evaluated with less risk. Indirect field tests of maximal aerobic power currently provide reliable and valid estimates of population averages.

IMPORTANT RESEARCH TOPICS

16. More research is needed to establish a firm relationship between cardiorespiratory fitness (maximal and submaximal factors) and various components of health.
17. Within the context of health-related fitness, more precise and valid tests of submaximal cardiorespiratory capacity are needed.

Metabolic Fitness

Metabolic fitness has been defined as resulting "from adequate hormonal actions, particularly for insulin, normal blood and tissue carbohydrate and lipid metabolism, and a favorable ratio of lipid to carbohydrate oxidized." It has been shown that various aspects of health are associated with glycemic status, lipid-lipoprotein profile, and the ratio of lipid to carbohydrate oxidation. It has also been shown that regular endurance training favorably affects these factors.

Although the concept of metabolic fitness makes intuitive sense, there is no consensus about a definition since this might include many other factors (e.g., other hormones and substrates). Nor do we know how all these factors should be measured and applied to health-related fitness. There are standardized procedures for measuring fasting blood glucose, glucose and insulin responses to a glucose load, and fasting blood lipid and lipoprotein profiles. However, there are no standardized tests that would evaluate the ratio of lipid to carbohydrate oxidation and allow its relevance to health to be studied.

IMPORTANT RESEARCH TOPICS

18. The conceptual definition of metabolic fitness should be clarified and extended.
19. Other physiological and biochemical factors which might be involved in metabolic fitness need to be explored.

Measurement of Health Status and Quality of Life

The careful study of physical activity and health requires precise measurement of both concepts. The measurement of health is complex, depending on the conceptual and pragmatic definition used. There are at least five facets of health, with potential for corresponding measures. A genetic facet governs basic health structure and influences the other four facets of health. Biochemical, physiologic, and morphologic conditions reflect a facet of health that determines disease, illness, organ impairment, disability, or handicap. A functional facet, closely related to this, includes the capacity to undertake the usual activities and requirements of daily life. Mental facets include mood and cognitive processes. The facet of health potential includes longevity, functional potential, and the extent of any disability. Measurement genres reflect these facets and include mortality, morbidity, risk factor prevalence, use of medical care, disability, physical function, mental function, functional activities, bodily well being, emotional well being, self-concept, global perceptions of health, and healthy life years. Physical activity impinges upon most of these facets and measures of health.

Measures of health status depend on the goals of the assessment and how one makes and uses the observations. The objective may be to evaluate or to predict health. Alternatively, there may be a wish to test the response to clinical interventions, health promotion efforts, or systems for the delivery of medical care. Such evaluations can stimulate economic, social, and political reform, but must consider changes in and vagaries of disease and health classification. Health status measures have to date tended to focus on disease events rather than individual health. However, individual measures, like health risk appraisals, can help to evaluate and encourage efforts at health promotion.

Traditional measures have focused on the absence of health. Mortality statistics take death as an end point and try to attribute specific causes of death. They can also project life expectancy at specified ages. Common measures of morbidity are disease incidence, case-fatality ratios, hospital admissions, bed-days, treatment costs, and lost days of work for specific causes. Morbidity and mortality statistics should separate disease events from measures of disease or illness burden like hospital days and treatment costs. However, combined morbidity and mortality measures like quality-adjusted life expectancy may be more use-

ful in evaluating program effectiveness. Medical care cost indicators reflect the economic burden of mortality, morbidity and other direct and indirect costs associated with specific diseases. International and intercultural comparisons of these and other measures of health status may be impeded by differences in classification schema, data collection procedures, and geopolitical circumstances, which may also change over time.

Because of the high costs of collecting and compiling data, morbidity statistics usually come from smaller, less representative samples than the total population. Errors in recording, classifying, or processing data limit the utility of morbidity and mortality statistics, and inevitably they do not reflect positive health status.

Problems in conceptualizing constructs, especially positive health status, have hindered the measurement of health. Moreover, inadequate data sources and resources have restricted the development of measures even when appropriate measurement concepts exist. Nonetheless, progress continues in the development of measures that reflect well-being and functioning. Well-being includes concepts like bodily well-being, emotional well-being, self-concept, and global perceptions of health. Functioning includes physical and cognitive functioning, and the capacity to perform both the discretionary and the essential activities of daily living. Investigators have used such population-based measures as two-week disability days, disability-free life expectancy, and psychological well-being as measures of the quality of life. Global health measures include healthy life expectancy or disability-free life expectancy. Such measures of positive health may be useful in international and intercultural comparisons. The availability of data for many measures is limited by the validity of the existing instruments and the capacity to reflect a simple summary score.

Different measures of health are appropriate to different age groups and to each sex to the extent that their sociologic, behavioral, and health concerns and needs differ. Morbidity and mortality statistics are more useful in reflecting the health status of older adult populations who are affected by a variety of chronic diseases. Estimated years of potential life lost can help to emphasize diseases that kill younger populations, especially where chronic disease morbidity or mortality are very low. Quality of life measures have proven valuable in reflecting the health status of older adults where functional impairment, morbidity and disability are commonplace. These measures may also be useful in reflecting the positive health of younger

age groups, even where morbidity, disability, and functional impairment are rare. However, quality of life measures suitable for younger populations are only starting to evolve.

IMPORTANT RESEARCH TOPICS

Because physical activity has an important influence on health, the following research recommendations apply to physical activity as it relates to the measurement of health. Each research recommendation reflects both generic as well as condition-specific health facets. They should focus on positive health. They should also represent the needs, interests, and special concerns of varying population subgroups, including children, women, older adults and the disadvantaged. Specifically, research efforts should include the following.

20. Develop reliable and valid measures that are sensitive to changes in individual and population health.
21. Develop outcome measures suitable for epidemiologic research, health promotion programs and preventive services, as well as composite measures for the assessment of functioning morbidity, mortality, and disability (e.g., quality adjusted life years).
22. Explore different methods of refining, weighing, and identifying the structure, utility, and preference of various health states in order to elucidate the meaning of composite health scores such as quality-adjusted life expectancy.

Chapter 5

Physical Activity, Fitness, and Health: Status and Determinants

Demography of Leisure-Time Physical Activity

Recent questionnaire surveys in Australia, Canada, and the United States suggest that about 40% of adults are active enough in their leisure-time to obtain a variety of health benefits. That is, they exercise regularly at activities of at least moderate intensity. Ten percent of adults in these countries report exercising at least three times weekly for 20 or more minutes at an intensity considered sufficient to develop and/or sustain cardiorespiratory fitness. Depending on how "sedentary" is defined, at least one third to one half of adults in these countries fall into this category.

In Australia, Canada, Finland, the former German Democratic Republic, and the United States, there has been a modest increase in the self-reported prevalence of healthful levels of exercise over at least the past decade. This increase does not extend to heavy exercise for all these countries. In Australia, there is some hint of a recent levelling off while heavy exercise has recently become less common in Canada.

Although good data on non-leisure activity are scarce, Finnish surveys show steadily decreasing occupational activity, including bicycling to work. This is probably typical of countries where increased exercise has been reported, but it is not possible to make any statements about long-term trends in total energy expenditure.

There is considerable consistency among nations in the relationship of self-reported, leisure-time, physical activity levels to sex, age, and education. Sex differences are minimal when exercise intensity is moderate or light, that is, males and females report spending about the same amount of time exercising. Male-female differences are most pronounced when the definition of "active" involves high-intensity exercise (except when "high intensity" is defined relative to capacity in a sex-specific manner). Males are, on average, 50% more likely to report being vigorously active than females. Women appear to have increased their overall

exercise levels more rapidly than men in the 1980s, but this is probably not true of vigorous exercise.

National surveys of physical activity consistently reveal that, by most definitions, including total active time or total energy expended per week, exercise prevalence declines steadily with age. When age-specific values for relative intensity are used as a means of defining vigorous activity, this trend disappears. The only population survey that included children and adolescents shows a precipitous drop in activity on leaving high school. Older adults increased their exercise levels more than younger ones during the 1980s.

Leisure-time physical activity is consistently more common among groups with more education. Recent surveys in Australia, Britain, Canada, and the United States all reveal that the most educated group is 50 to 200% more likely than the least educated group to undertake deliberate exercise. There is mixed evidence as to the fate of the education gap over the recent past. Canadian data show a modest narrowing of the gap from 1981 to 1988, whereas a slight widening was found in the United States for the period 1986 to 1990.

IMPORTANT RESEARCH TOPICS

23. Further monitoring of leisure-time activity in adult populations is needed to identify (a) whether the prevalence of exercise is still increasing, and (b) if women, older adults, and less educated groups are closing the gap by becoming more active more quickly than the rest of the population.

24. New studies are required to determine (a) if other countries, including less industrialized countries, have similar activity levels, and (b) if occupational demands and other sources of physical activity are diminishing as suspected.

25. Better data are needed on people with low levels of activity, children, and older

adults and on forms of physical activity other than deliberate exercise (occupational activity, personal transportation, household chores). Customarily-used questionnaire methods will have to be adapted for these purposes.

26. Population surveys should provide sufficient detail on activity type, intensity, frequency, duration, seasonality, and social context to permit investigation of exercise stimuli and dosages relevant to all dimensions of health-related fitness. Guidelines are needed to develop the questionnaires for such surveys.

27. Definitions of exercise dose should be standardized with respect to intensity, frequency, and duration. When relative intensity is used, age- and sex-related adjustments should be consistently applied, and should be based on better data than are currently available.

Determinants of Participation in Physical Activity

As the health consequences of physical activity and inactivity become better documented, it becomes more important to understand the factors that influence participation in active leisure behavior (exercise). These influences, often termed "determinants," can be categorized as personal attributes, environmental characteristics, and features of the physical activity itself.

Though most studies prior to 1988 were conducted on non-representative samples, two-thirds of the more recent studies have employed community samples. Therefore, their findings should be more widely generalizable than earlier results, at least to "whites" from North America and Australia. Whereas earlier studies had focused on men, two thirds of the studies currently reviewed had women and men as subjects. Previous reviews had called for prospective studies, and half of the studies currently reviewed had follow-ups ranging from 7 weeks to 15 years. The continuing shortcomings are the emphasis on maintenance and dropout rather than adoption of exercise, and the restriction to vigorous exercise rather than including lower intensity activities.

Demographic variables continue to be among the most consistent and strongest correlates of vigorous exercise. In general, younger, male, well-educated, and, in North America, non-hispanic,

"white" subgroups tend to be more active than others. Contrary to popular belief, there is little relationship between exercise patterns during youth, obesity, or smoking, and adult exercise habits. Self-efficacy, self-schemata, expectation of benefits, intention to exercise, and barriers are generally related to exercise participation, while attitudes and knowledge are not. In cross-sectional and prospective studies, social factors, especially specific social support for exercise, are usually significant correlates of exercise behavior. Few physical environment variables have been studied, but objectively measured access to facilities is related to participation in formal exercise programs. Both the intensity and the perceived effort of exercise are negatively correlated with participation. These findings suggest that most people prefer lower intensity activities.

Consistent associations were found in every category of determinants. These findings emphasize the importance of viewing exercise behavior as being influenced by many personal and environmental forces.

Twenty recent studies were reviewed. They represent methodological advances over the interventions reviewed for the 1988 consensus. Internal validity and generalizability have improved. Prior to 1988, most intervention studies used uncontrolled case and cohort designs. Since 1988, more than half the studies have used randomized or quasi-experimental designs, including large samples of males and females of various ages. A few studies of ethnic and minority groups have appeared, but such studies have largely been limited to the United States.

The existing literature permits the following conclusions regarding interventions designed to increase exercise participation.

1. Educational counseling and behavior modification or cognitive-behavior modification principles can be implemented with exercise programs. They are generally accompanied by an increased frequency of exercise or of the time spent in exercising at least for the limited periods of observation (typically 4 to 20 weeks).

2. With the exception of studies closely linked with onsite programs or periodic supervision (e.g., work site, clinics, or schools), the studies do not demonstrate that either exercise intensity or the total volume of daily physical activity has been increased enough to improve physical fitness, or to reduce the risk of future morbidity or mortality.

3. Most studies have used either indirect measures of exercise behavior (e.g., self-reports) or

simple measures of physical fitness, based on heart rate or treadmill time. The absence of uniform outcome measures prevents a clear comparison of results across studies.

4. Most interventions have not been based on a broader theoretical model of behavioral change, such as stage theories, nor have they considered overall activity history or the companion literature on the determinants of exercise behavior.

Interventions, regardless of type, are usually associated with moderate increases in the frequency of exercising. An increase in adherence success from about 4 in 10 participants without intervention, to about 6 in 10 participants following intervention, is typical. The superiority of behavior change interventions versus a reduction in the intensity, duration, and frequency of the usual prescriptions used for increasing physical fitness merits direct testing.

Increases in physical activity or fitness associated with the interventions diminished as follow-up time increased. Few comparisons have used an attention-control condition. Therefore, generalizations about the effectiveness of specific components of the interventions for specific populations are not possible.

Although there have been too few studies since 1988 to permit meaningful clustering of effect sizes according to other important characteristics of the studies, it appears that the size of the intervention effects reported has been inversely related to the scientific quality of the studies.

IMPORTANT RESEARCH TOPICS

28. Research on determinants should focus on personal and environmental variables that can be manipulated and applied in interventions. When feasible, findings from observational studies need to be verified by experimental research. Genetic and biological factors influencing exercise behavior also need to be understood.

29. Determinants, and their relative importance, are likely to vary for different populations, population subgroups, and cultures. These differences need to be investigated. What are the similarities and differences in the determinants of exercise behavior for men and women, and for peoples of different ages, ethnic groups, education, and geographic locations?

30. More and better studies of the determinants of various dimensions of exercise behavior, particularly different intensities and types, including sedentary behaviors, are needed.

31. More studies of the determinants of the adoption of regular exercise are needed. Continued study of adherence, long-term maintenance, and relapse is also recommended.

32. Studies should use valid measures of physical activity as well as valid measures of potential determinants that are comparable across studies. Objective measures of environmental determinants should be developed.

33. The primary need is for the development and evaluation of efficacious approaches that encourage the adoption and long-term maintenance of exercise behavior. Personal, environmental, and exercise characteristics reported as important in observational studies should be targeted in intervention research. Interventions probably require tailoring to specific populations, subpopulations, and cultures, but the means of tailoring are as yet not well developed. Face-to-face interventions, suited to clinically-based applications, should be compared with mediated interventions (e.g., television, telephone, and mail) suited for large-scale population-interventions to determine their relative effectiveness. Methods for documenting and improving the quality of intervention (e.g., program leadership) should be studied.

34. Interventions have disproportionately emphasized a change of personal attributes (e.g., attitudes, intentions, and self-efficacy) among exercise participants, but the efficacy of the interventions which have been used in attempts to change these psychological attributes has not been established. There is a need to evaluate interventions that target variables in the social and physical environments.

35. There is a need to develop valid measures for assessing the rewarding experiences and outcomes of exercise participation that can reinforce participation and minimize the likelihood of relapse to sedentary habits.

36. There is a need to determine the types, intensities, durations, locations, social settings and times of exercise that maximize the likelihood of its adoption and maintenance.

37. There is a need to standardize, or to reconcile, different measures of exercise behavior.

Assessing Population Levels of Health-Related Fitness: Methodological Concerns

Demographic studies within populations have yielded useful information on growth, aging, and sex-related differences of health-related fitness. Effects of socio-economic status and overall lifestyle have also been demonstrated, and associations between individual markers of fitness have been explored. However, the interpretation of demographic data is currently hampered. Key considerations include the following:

- Whether the samples of subjects tested are representative of the populations under discussion.
- The extent of allowance for specific factors that distort cross-sectional survey results.
- The ability to counter the problems that develop when longitudinal observations are collected over several decades.
- The severe technical constraints that are imposed by measurement techniques appropriate to large-scale surveys.
- The interactive impact of such surveys upon population fitness and health.

In terms of sampling, a large proportion of data has been obtained on convenience samples. Because of barriers such as geography and language, even entire communities may be representative only of themselves. In larger communities, data may be restricted to those born in a single year, with complications from cohort effects. Relatively few investigators have attempted to collect data on stratified random samples of national populations. Such information becomes heavily distorted because a high proportion of older individuals are excluded from the evaluation.

Even if large samples are recruited, the results of cross-sectional surveys are affected by climatic factors, selective migration, intercurrent patholo-

gies, and differences in the life experience of various age cohorts. Seasonal factors, once recognized, are readily countered by spreading observations randomly over the entire year. The problem of chronic disease becomes widespread in older segments of most communities, complicating comparisons of data both within and between populations. Activity patterns, nutrition and lifestyle differ between age-cohorts in many communities, further limiting the potential for meaningful comparisons.

Longitudinal surveys do not resolve all technical difficulties. The constancy of methodology and of subjective responses to testing must be assured. The effects of aging tend to become confounded with secular trends in community behavior, and except in isolated communities, sample attrition is a major problem. Currently, the ideal approach is a mixed cross-sectional/longitudinal design.

International standardization of methodology has rarely been applied in interpopulation comparisons. Occasional surveys have applied high technology methodology to large populations, but usually the interpretation of data is complicated by the use of very simple test procedures that lack a strong relationship to health-related fitness.

Intrapopulation comparisons commonly examine effects of age, sex, socio-economic factors, activity patterns, and overall lifestyle. Sampling problems are less critical when making comparisons within a given population. However, whether comparing men to women, or children of various ages, there remains a critical need for agreement on methods of allowing for interindividual differences in body size. Gender-related differences also become confounded with cultural influences. Probably because of methodological problems, large-scale surveys show surprisingly little influence of reported activity upon estimates of fitness. Likewise, the observed relationship between fitness and other facets of lifestyle has been quite limited. On the other hand, there are substantial differences of activity patterns related to socio-economic status.

Interpopulation comparisons are currently severely limited by the lack of representative data. Body mass for height appears to be substantially lower in many of the economically poorer countries, and such regions generally show health advantages in terms of blood pressure and serum cholesterol. However, if aerobic power is expressed in ml/(kg × min), there are surprisingly few differences among different countries.

The challenges to future investigators are to adopt more appropriate sampling techniques, to devise methodology that remains valid within the context of a large survey, and to establish dose/response relationships that will enable a definition of clinically significant interpopulation differences in the variables under examination.

IMPORTANT RESEARCH TOPICS

38. Sampling techniques—there is a pressing need to develop better recruitment methods to reduce the response bias inherent in most current population studies, particularly the underrecruitment of older individuals and those from lower socioeconomic strata.
39. Choice of criteria for population health—should we be concerned with the mean level of fitness reached by a given population or with the proportion of that population who fail to meet a certain minimum standard on selected variables?
40. Significant fitness levels—populations may score well on one criterion, but poorly on another. Thus, in assessing interpopulation differences, there is a need to identify which are the most important components of fitness from the viewpoint of health. It will be necessary to determine how these variables interact with each other, and to develop accurate and internationally standardized techniques for the assessment of such fitness on samples of population.
41. Significant covariates—in assessing the impact of fitness levels upon health, it is necessary to develop and to use simple, standardized techniques to assess important covariates such as cigarette smoking, nutrition and exposure to air pollutants.
42. There remains a need to carry out well-controlled interpopulation comparisons of health-related fitness, using standardized techniques.

Physical Activity, Nutrition, Fitness, and Health

Physical activity increases the utilization of many nutrients. The ability to perform vigorous exercise depends on the replacement of these nutrients through diet. Of particular concern are the nutrients used as fuel and water. Other nutrients are also of interest, such as the vitamins used during fuel oxidation, and the vitamins and minerals necessary for oxygen transport and protection against increased oxygen flux. However, much misinformation is currently purveyed to the public regarding the need for special ergogenic aids at all levels of exercise, and such misinformation should be countered.

Lipids and carbohydrates are normally the main sources of food energy. A small carbohydrate intake seems sufficient to allow a complete oxidation of lipids without detrimental ketone body production. Prolonged aerobic exercise induces an increase in carbohydrate utilization and a depletion of carbohydrate stores; the latter effect is associated with an increase in postexercise lipid oxidation. The enzymatic adaptations observed after exercise favor glycogen resynthesis, which is maximized by the ingestion of a high carbohydrate diet. Under high-fat diet conditions, the body still gives a priority to the restoration of carbohydrate reserves. The notion that glucose or sugar feeding during the hour before exercise induces an insulin hypoglycemia, and thus increases glycogen use at the beginning of exercise, remains controversial. Moreover, there is little support for the idea that such a practice impairs endurance capacity.

A minimal lipid intake is necessary to supply the body with essential fatty acids. Current dietary recommendations assure sufficient levels of essential fatty acids but avoid an excessive lipid intake, thus minimizing the risks of cardiovascular disease, cancer, and obesity. These recommendations apply to both inactive and exercising persons.

Research indicates that amino acids provide not more than 5 to 15% of the total energy expended during exercise. However, the magnitude of this increased utilization leads to only a slight increase in protein needs with strenuous physical activity. Given an adequate mixed diet, the slight increase has little consequence for fitness and health. Most people in most countries report consuming over twice the quantity of protein recommended daily for sedentary individuals, leaving more than adequate margin to cover any slight increase of needs with physical activity and tissue hypertrophy. Of concern may be the individual who combines a low energy intake with an increased protein requirement. Supplemental protein and individual amino acids, if they have any effect, act by adding energy to the system.

The increased energy output accompanying physical activity is important in controlling body mass. However, the ability of exercise to induce an energy deficit depends also on the adjustment of postexercise energy intake, and possible adaptive changes in resting metabolic rate.

Exercise increases body heat production. Heat is partly removed from the body by the evaporation of water, thus fluid replenishment is necessary if plasma volume and the ability to thermoregulate are to be maintained. Unfortunately, the thirst mechanism is usually inadequate to ensure *ad libitum* replacement of losses. Of particular concern are individuals exercising in the heat (where fluid losses may be great), and the elderly (in whom the thirst mechanism is diminished). Replenishment may be adequately accomplished with water under most circumstances.

Vitamins and minerals are essential to health. There is no clear evidence to suggest increased needs for the majority of these nutrients arise from physical activity. Zinc, copper, and chromium are of particular concern, however, because the intake of these nutrients by the general population is below present recommended dietary allowance. Cumulative losses in sweat, at least in the case of zinc and copper, can be significant. With the concern over increased free-radical production during exercise, there is a growing interest in the possible role of the antioxidants (e.g., vitamins C and E) in preserving fitness and health. However, there is insufficient research to draw conclusions at this time. Supplementation of iron and calcium may be of some benefit for some women. Interactions of trace minerals may result in a precipitation of deficiencies if intakes are imbalanced. A diet designed to promote overall health should be sufficient to cover needs of physical activity without supplementation, provided energy requirements are met.

IMPORTANT RESEARCH TOPICS

---

43. What are the mechanisms by which exercise can increase postexercise energy intake and expenditure, and what is the contribution of increases in postexercise energy intake and expenditure to the potential energy deficit induced by exercise?

44. Does exercise affect the minimal requirements of carbohydrate and lipids?

45. Does exercise have an effect on macronutrient preference (e.g., carbohydrate)?

46. Does exercise affect the need for micronutrients (e.g., chromium)?

47. What is the best way to replenish fluid during and after exercise—with water alone or in conjunction with carbohydrate and/or electrolytes?

48. Do nutrient needs with exercise change across various segments of the population at various ages?

49. Does the supplementation of protein to levels of ≥ 2.0 g/day per kg of body weight enhance the increase in fat-free mass associated with resistance training? If so, will the increase in fat-free mass be reflected by an increased resting metabolic rate which could facilitate fat loss?

50. Will the supplementation of calcium in combination with resistance and aerobic exercise training reduce bone mineral losses in young amenorrheic and postmenopausal women with aging?

Adjuvants to Physical Activity

Adjuvants to physical activity are defined as those measures or practices which, because of their potential physiological effects, are used in the hope of enhancing the benefits or reducing the potential detrimental effects of physical activity on fitness and health. Although there are many measures or practices that could be discussed, this statement focuses on electrical stimulation, massage, sauna, sudation garments, and questionable exercise devices.

Electrical Stimulation

Electrical stimulation increases isometric strength and isokinetic strength at both slow and fast contraction speeds. The magnitude of these effects is inversely related to the initial muscle strength of the individual. There seems to be no effect on muscular endurance. Contrary to ordinary strength training, electrical stimulation probably activates Type II better than Type I muscle fibers. In patients, these effects may translate to improved functional status. Electrical stimulation may alleviate postoperative pain, enabling the patient to conduct muscular training more effectively. Thus, electrical stimulation is a well-founded adjuvant to muscle training in the rehabilitation of injured (e.g., knee-operated) exercise participants and patients with neurological disorders, but it does not seem to give any extra benefit over equivalent voluntary training of healthy individuals.

Massage

Massage is widely and increasingly used with several intents, such as to enhance muscular relaxation and joint mobility prior to exercise; to prevent and alleviate muscular cramps, soreness, and pain; to hasten recovery after strenuous efforts; and to speed up the healing of soft tissue injuries, thereby restoring flexibility and joint mobility. These benefits are expected on the basis of the alleged physiological effects of massage.

A large proportion of exercise participants and patients receiving massage perceive its effects to be positive and useful, but this could be in part due to nonspecific placebo effects. However, massage has specific physiological effects, decreasing alpha motorneuron excitability, slightly increasing the range of motion in some joints, and slightly increasing the cutaneous and muscle blood flow. The practical significance of these effects remains to be proven. Recent studies have not shown massage to cause changes in serum beta-endorphins, muscle strength, circulatory responses to submaximal exercise, or short-term recovery from intense muscular activity. In conclusion, the physiological effects and preventive, therapeutic, and restorative efficacy of massage have been inadequately studied. Therefore, the use of massage as an adjuvant to exercise has to be considered at present as mainly "educated empiricism."

Sauna

Sauna has been suggested for numerous purposes including warming-up before training and competition, mental and physical relaxation before and after training and competition, facilitation of mental and physical recovery, weight reduction, prevention and treatment of musculoskeletal injuries, prevention of respiratory infections, training of the circulatory system and autonomous regulation, as well as acclimation to heat. Most of these proposed benefits are based more on perceived effects, reasoning, and indirect evidence than on well-conducted research.

On the basis of proven physiological effects, sauna has been used to reduce fluid loss and thus an acute weight reduction on certain types of athletes, for neuromuscular relaxation, and for heat acclimation. However, the temporary impairment of fluid and electrolyte balance, and of motivation for all-out effort that are caused by especially intensive bathing, as well as practical problems of environmental control, considerably limit the use of sauna. Favorable psychosomatic effects like stimulation-relaxation, facilitation of recovery from strenuous effort, and decreased postexercise musculoskeletal symptoms are commonly experienced among frequent sauna users. On the other hand, sauna bathing is not an efficient stimulus or substitute for circulatory training. Furthermore, intensive sauna bathing, or sauna followed by sudden cold exposure (e.g., a plunge into a cold lake or a shower), may increase the risk of cardiovascular complications and thermal injury. The risks are probably greater under certain conditions and in certain populations (e.g., infrequent use, pregnancy, cardiovascular disease, elderly).

Sudation (Sweat-Inducing) Garments

Sudation garments are used to create a temporary hot microclimate by preventing evaporative heat loss. Their intent is to enhance exercise-heat tolerance, and thus the person's performance capacity in hot climates. The few, but well-conducted studies specifically addressing this problem indicate that, at least in well-trained subjects, training in sudation garments does not offer significant advantages over training in ordinary exercise clothing. Neither increase exercise heat tolerance as much as training in warm conditions. This finding, and the extra physical and perceived demands of wearing sudation garments during training, do not support their use as a means to enhance exercise-heat tolerance.

Sudation garments are used to enhance the temporary weight loss induced by sweating. An increase of skin and deep body temperatures offers a strong stimulus for sweating. Skin and deep body temperature and sweating all increase more when the same exercise is performed in sudation garments rather than ordinary training clothing. Thus, exercise in a sudation garment enhances the acute weight reduction, or causes an equivalent weight reduction for less energy expenditure. From a practical point of view, the extra physical and perceived demands of using sudation garments, and the negative impact of fluid and electrolyte losses on physical performance capacity, limit the usefulness of sudation garments as a means of achieving an acute weight reduction. Hyperthermia, dehydration, and thermal injury can all result from the use of sudation garments.

Selected Exercise Devices

There are many exercise devices which have proven beneficial effects upon fitness and health (e.g., treadmills, cycle ergometers, resistance equipment). However, there are also many very questionable commercial exercise devices (e.g., bust developers and vibrating machines) that have no apparent scientific rationale. Most of these devices are associated with the multi-billion dollar weight-loss and figure-control industry. Some are passive devices that require no exertion or additional energy expenditure on the part of the user. Others include active movement, but the claims by each for spot reduction or figure enhancement are unfounded.

Unfortunately, few research studies have examined the efficacy of exercise devices that fall into the "questionable" category. In most cases, claims are made without supporting research data, and the scientific community expresses its skepticism on the basis of an evaluation of these claims against established scientific fact. Where actual scientific studies have been conducted, the resulting data generally do not support the manufacturer's claims. In some cases, manufacturers have been successfully prosecuted for fraudulent claims.

IMPORTANT RESEARCH TOPICS

51. What is the physiological basis for the muscle strengthening that is associated with neuromuscular electrical stimulation, for example, functional overload of Type I fibers (as in voluntary contraction), or preferential Type II fiber recruitment based on the specific characteristics of electrical stimulation?

52. What are the structural and functional effects in muscles, ligaments, and tendons of different types of massage after strenuous exercise and in post-injury rehabilitation?

53. The potential therapeutic and restorative benefits of sauna bathing for health and fitness should be further investigated.

54. Since many of the proposed adjuvants to physical activity are used for the purposes of inducing weight loss or reshaping the body figure, are there adjuvants that might work synergistically with physical activity to produce long-term changes in metabolic rate? Agents that increase sympathetic activity or body temperature would be likely candidates.

Chapter 6

Human Adaptation to Acute and Chronic Physical Activity

Physical Activity and the Cardiovascular System

The acute response to muscular exercise provides the greatest challenge to the cardiovascular system, demanding a complex integration of the local regulation of blood flow to the active skeletal muscle and neural regulation of the hemodynamic response. In sustained dynamic exercise, the active muscle must receive a blood flow appropriate to its increased metabolic needs, and at the same time the brain and heart must receive an adequate blood flow to maintain their normal functions. In static exercise, the mechanical obstruction to skeletal muscle blood flow caused by increased intramuscular pressure opposes effects from the local dilation of the resistance vessels.

During intense dynamic exercise, there is a marked increase in oxygen delivery to the muscles; this is accomplished by an increase in heart rate, stroke volume, and total body arterio-venous oxygen difference. However, there is only a small increase in mean arterial pressure, and peripheral vascular resistance is markedly decreased. Vasodilation in the resistance vessels of the active skeletal muscle can increase local blood flow to 250-300 ml/100g of muscle/minute, explaining the marked decrease in peripheral vascular resistance. The underlying mechanism is not known; however, many metabolic stimuli have been suggested. During dynamic exercise involving a large proportion of the skeletal muscle mass, the ability to increase cardiac output, and thereby maintain mean arterial blood pressure, is the factor limiting maximal oxygen uptake.

During "static" exercise with contractions of the skeletal muscle maintained at approximately 30 to 50% of the maximal voluntary force, there is little increase in oxygen consumption, a moderate increase in cardiac output and heart rate, and no change in stroke volume. Total peripheral vascular resistance remains relatively constant, with a marked increase in mean arterial blood pressure.

Both dynamic and static exercise lead to increased activity of the sympathetic nervous system and decreased activity of the parasympathetic nervous system. Two neural mechanisms are responsible: central neural mechanism ("central command") and a reflex mechanism ("exercise pressor reflex"). The exercise pressor reflex is mediated by Group III muscle afferents, which respond mainly to mechanical perturbations, and Group IV muscle afferents, which respond mainly to metabolic changes in the contracting skeletal muscle. The arterial baroreceptors, cardiopulmonary receptors, and the reflexes that they mediate also appear to be involved in the control of blood pressure during exercise.

Metabolites and other substances produced in active skeletal muscle have three major roles in orchestrating the cardiovascular response: (a) to act locally in causing vasodilation of the resistance vessels; (b) to activate sensory receptors in skeletal muscle which reflexly excite medullary cardiovascular control areas via Group IV afferent nerve fibers, thereby increasing sympathetic neuronal outflow to the heart and blood vessels; and (c) to modulate the sympathetic control of the resistance vessels in the active skeletal muscle.

The chronic adaptation of the cardiovascular system to repeated bouts of muscular exercise depends on the type and intensity of the activity that has been undertaken. Dynamic exercise training leads to an increase in maximal oxygen uptake, due to an enhanced ability to increase stroke volume and to widen the total body arterio-venous oxygen difference. The ability to deliver a greater peak stroke volume may reflect an eccentric hypertrophy of the left ventricle rather than an increase in the contractile state. Other results of dynamic exercise include increases in total blood volume, vascular capacitance, venous compliance, vascular reactivity to receptor agonists, and decreased afterloading. These changes affect cardiovascular regulation and may contribute to orthostatic intolerance.

With static exercise training, there is no appreciable increase in maximal oxygen uptake. However, eccentric hypertrophy of the left ventricle can again develop, increasing the ability to deliver the same stroke volume against a markedly increased mean arterial pressure (afterload).

IMPORTANT RESEARCH TOPICS

55. What is the local mechanism causing vasodilation in the resistance vessels of exercising skeletal muscle?
56. How is the metabolic demand in contracting skeletal muscle sensed and how does it affect the cardiovascular response?
57. Is there a change in sympathetic outflow to exercising skeletal muscle with training, and if so, what is its effect?
58. What is the relative importance of central command and the exercise pressor reflex in matching the cardiovascular response to the type and intensity of exercise, and how are the two mechanisms integrated?
59. What are the factors limiting maximal oxygen intake in different physiological and pathophysiological conditions?
60. What is the effect of gender and age on the acute cardiovascular response and adaptation to exercise?

Physical Activity and the Microcirculation of Cardiac and Skeletal Muscle

Exercise training increases the capacity of the cardiovascular system to transport nutrients to active skeletal muscle tissue. The increased vascular transport capacity makes possible an enhanced peak rate of oxidative metabolism in active muscles. Aerobic training increases the vascular transport capacity in both cardiac and skeletal muscle by augmenting both the peak blood flow and capillary exchange capacity. The increases in transport capacity result from both structural adaptations and altered control of vascular resistance. Structural vascular adaptations take at least two forms: increases in the cross-sectional area and length of the large and small arteries and veins (i.e., vascular growth) and increased numbers of capillaries (and other microvessels) per gram of muscle (i.e., angiogenesis).

Vascular adaptation induced by endurance exercise training develops relatively uniformly throughout the myocardium, whereas it seems less uniformly distributed in skeletal muscle. Increased capillary density and increased vascular transport capacity occur around muscle fibers that experience the largest increase in activity during exercise. However, vascular adaptation may not be heterogenous in the skeletal muscle of all species.

Angiogenesis has been demonstrated in the coronary circulation; endurance exercise training causes moderate cardiac hypertrophy, while maintaining or increasing the capillary density and increasing the arteriolar density. Changes in coronary vascular control induced by endurance exercise training include altered coronary responses to vasoactive substances, changes in endothelium-mediated vasoregulation, and alterations in the cellular-molecular control of intracellular free Ca^{2+} in both endothelial and vascular smooth muscle cells.

IMPORTANT RESEARCH TOPICS

61. There is a need for anatomical data, describing the effects of exercise training on small arteries, arterioles, venules, and small veins, in order to understand structural vascular adaptation and vascular remodeling.
62. The hypothesis that structural and functional vascular adaptations occur around muscle fibers that experience the greatest relative increase in activity during training bouts needs to be tested systematically in humans.
63. The hypothesis that exercise training induces changes in local control of microvascular resistance must be tested in both skeletal and cardiac muscles.
64. The interactions of microvascular adaptations induced by exercise training with disease states such as atherosclerosis, hypertension, and diabetes require elucidation.
65. The effects of weight training on skeletal muscle microvascular beds also require further investigation.
66. The signal or signals initiating structural and functional adaptive responses should be defined.

Physical Activity and the Pulmonary System

The responses to exercise in the young untrained healthy pulmonary system [$\dot{V}O_2$max < 50-55 ml/

(kg × min)] can be summarized as follows: the alveolar to arterial oxygen partial pressure difference widens two- to three-fold during maximal exercise, due primarily to an increased nonuniformity in distribution of alveolar ventilation relative to pulmonary capillary flow. Expiratory air flow is rarely limited significantly by airway collapse. The transpulmonary pressure developed by the inspiratory muscles reaches about 50% of their dynamic capacity. A significant compensatory but highly variable hyperventilatory response to heavy and maximum exercise occurs in all healthy untrained subjects (decrease in partial pressure of CO_2 in arterial blood 5 to 15 Torr). Based on voluntary mimicking of the exercise pleural pressure volume loop, the oxygen cost of hyperpnea is estimated to average 8-10% of $\dot{V}O_2max$ in subjects who require maximal ventilation in the range of 100 to 130 l/min. In long-term, heavy endurance exercise, breathing frequency and ventilatory output gradually rise. Dead space ventilation also rises, but alveolar ventilation remains adequate. At very heavy sustained work rates (> 85% $\dot{V}O_2max$) significant diaphragmatic fatigue occurs.

Adaptation of the healthy pulmonary system to the "training stimulus" may be summarized as follows: total lung capacity and its subdivisions do not change more than a few percent with prolonged, general physical training. Reported differences in some highly trained athletes, young or old, are most likely the result of pre-selection. Phylogenic differences in highly fit versus sedentary species show that the lung lacks adaptability compared to the highly adaptable structural capacities of muscle mitochondria, muscle capillaries, and heart muscle mitochondria. The diaphragm at all ages is adaptable to whole body physical training in terms of changes in aerobic capacity and perhaps even in fiber type.

Demand versus capacity in the highly fit, healthy pulmonary system may be described as follows. Diffusion limitation for oxygen at the alveolar capillary level becomes significant and arterial hypoxemia occurs as the increase in pulmonary blood flow exceeds the individual's ability to expand the pulmonary capillary blood volume. If the respiratory minute volume exceeds 150 to 160 l/min, the expiratory flow rate becomes limited by airway collapse, inspiratory muscles develop more than 90% of their maximal available pressure, and ventilation is mechanically limited. In such circumstances, the local oxygen consumption of the respiratory muscles will exceed 400 ml/min or 15% of $\dot{V}O_2max$. With endurance exercise in excess of 85% of $\dot{V}O_2max$, significant diaphragmatic fatigue

occurs. The elastic recoil of the lung diminishes with normal aging, even in the non-smoking healthy human. Expiratory flow limitation is then reached even at moderate work rates, the functional residual capacity reaches resting levels or above, and the oxygen cost of exercise hyperpnea is increased relative to younger subjects.

The role of pulmonary system is a limiting factor to $\dot{V}O_2max$ and endurance exercise performance in the following fashion. In the young untrained or moderately trained human with a $\dot{V}O_2max \leq$ 55 ml/(kg × min) or a peak respiratory minute volume < 120 l/min, diffusion limitation does not occur and the oxygen cost of breathing is not high enough to influence the ventilatory response significantly. In such subjects $\dot{V}O_2max$ or endurance performance is not determined to any significant extent by limitations of the lung and chest wall. At $\dot{V}O_2max \geq 65$ ml/(kg × min), an appreciable number of subjects will experience a significant limitation of $\dot{V}O_2max$ because of arterial oxyhemoglobin desaturation. The extent of this limitation is equivalent to at most 10 to 15% of $\dot{V}O_2max$. In highly fit humans with a peak respiratory minute volume in excess of 140 to 150 l/min, the oxygen cost of maximum ventilation will likely limit endurance performance significantly.

Several mechanisms responsible for the regulation of exercise hyperpnea have been identified in isolation. These include: (a) descending neural influences from higher locomotor areas of the central nervous system; (b) ascending neural signals from locomotor muscles initiated by mechanical and/or chemical changes in the locomotor muscles; and (c) humoral stimuli, including "CO_2 flow" to the lung.

The hyperventilatory response to heavy exercise is not yet accounted for. It remains correlated with increases in circulatory mediators from working muscle, including [H+], K+, norepinephrine and NH_3. Primary receptors and sensory pathways for transduction of the stimulus are controversial. Some of these same humoral stimuli change with duration of heavy exercise and have been implicated, along with body temperature, as potential mediators of the "tachypneic drift" during prolonged exercise. Regulation of upper airway calibre, respiratory muscle recruitment, and breathing pattern appear to optimize work of breathing during exercise.

IMPORTANT RESEARCH TOPICS

67. The relative contributions of basic neural and humoral control mechanisms to

exercise hyperpnea and hyperventilation need quantification.

68. The contribution of the respiratory muscles of the chest wall and abdomen to exercise hyperpnea and the mechanisms which regulate the specific recruitment of these muscles need detailed study.

69. It is unclear whether there is an accumulation of extravascular lung fluid at high levels of exercise. New techniques are needed to measure pulmonary extravascular fluid.

70. What factors cause maldistribution of alveolar ventilation, pulmonary capillary flow, and the ratio of alveolar ventilation to pulmonary capillary flow during heavy exercise?

71. How do pulmonary and cardiovascular control systems interact during exercise to regulate efferent sympathetic nervous activity and peripheral vascular resistance?

72. Longitudinal studies are needed to examine the adaptability of the pulmonary system to physical training in humans. Important issues include: effects on the strength and endurance of the respiratory muscles, the importance of maturation and aging on any local training "effect," and the effects upon the morphology of the lungs and chest wall.

Physical Activity and Hormonal Adaptation

Exercise requires major metabolic and cardiovascular adjustments to increase the supply of oxygen and fuels to the working muscles, while maintaining homeostasis. Changes in autonomic nervous activity and in hormone secretion help to accomplish these adjustments. Although the endocrine glands are the main source of hormones, a sharp distinction between the nervous and endocrine systems is no longer appropriate, because substances previously considered hormones may be released from nerves (e.g., gastrin), and neurotransmitters may spillover into the blood and act as hormones (e.g., norepinephrine). Changes in effective plasma hormone concentrations may be due to changes in secretion, plasma volume, binding, and/or clearance.

A single bout of exercise increases plasma concentrations of a large variety of hormones and decreases concentrations of only a few hormones. Although only studied for some hormones, the general impression is that the large changes in plasma concentrations of amine and peptide hormones seen during exercise result mainly from changes in secretion rate rather than changes in the rate of clearance. However, the clearance of hormones degraded primarily in the liver (e.g., the steroid hormones) may be expected to decrease during exercise, as splanchnic blood flow decreases.

A key role in the neuro-endocrine response to exercise is an increase of sympatho-adrenal activity and a resultant suppression of insulin secretion. These responses have major effects on metabolism and circulatory regulation, facilitating fuel supply and utilization. Increased plasma concentrations of certain hormones also affect metabolism (glucagon, growth hormone, cortisol) and fluid balance (renin, angiotensin, aldosterone, atrial natriuretic factor, vasopression). The signals eliciting changes in secretion of these hormones seem to include both *feedforward* and *feedback* regulatory mechanisms.

Hormonal responses to exercise are changed by endurance training, and the resting concentrations of some hormones may also be changed. In general, the hormonal response to a given absolute work rate is lessened after endurance training. However, the hormonal response to exercise at a given relative submaximal load is unchanged. During high intensity or maximal exercise, the response of the glucoregulatory hormones may be unchanged or even accentuated in the trained individual.

Changes in plasma catecholamine concentrations may be one of the mechanisms whereby aerobic training decreases resting arterial blood pressure. Whether resting plasma concentrations of catecholamines change with training remains controversial.

In both cross-sectional and longitudinal studies, training is associated with a lower post-absorptive concentration of insulin than that seen in untrained subjects. Although effects of training on gonadal function are unknown, intense endurance training has been associated with a reduction in plasma gonadal steroid concentrations in both women and men, namely decreased levels of estradiol and progesterone in women and testosterone in men. These gonadal steroidal changes may be associated with an impairment in pituitary luteinising hormone pulsatility.

Training-related changes in neuro-endocrine activity are often accompanied by changes in target tissue sensitivity and/or responsiveness. For instance, the responsiveness of adipose tissue lipolysis to catecholamines is increased by training, and insulin sensitivity is increased in trained subjects compared with untrained individuals. These changes in target tissue sensitivity more or less offset any effect of lower hormone concentrations in submaximal exercise and offer the possibility of increased maximal responsiveness to a physiological challenge. The major part of these adaptations occurs and disappears within a few days to a few weeks of beginning and ending training, respectively.

Mechanisms behind the changes in hormone concentrations and target tissue sensitivity with training are still not known. In vitro studies demonstrate that muscle contractions alone can enhance hormone sensitivity of muscle but changes in nonmuscle tissues (e.g., adipose tissue) also occur.

IMPORTANT RESEARCH TOPICS

73. There is a need to identify the signals and to determine the relative roles of feedforward versus feedback in controlling hormone secretion during exercise. The effects of training on these variables should also be studied.
74. The mechanisms involved in the adaptation of target tissues to exercise training need elucidation.
75. Possible interactive effects of diet and training on changes in hormone secretion and target tissue adaptations should be explored.
76. The effects of environment, gender, and genetic variation on hormone secretion and target tissue adaptations should be examined.

Physical Activity and Skeletal Muscle

Contractions of skeletal muscles provide the basis for all physical activities. Force is developed during an isometric contraction, whereas when muscle fibers shorten or lengthen, power (force × velocity) is produced or absorbed, respectively. Disuse, trauma, or disease each impair the ability of skeletal muscles to develop and sustain force and power and therefore decrease physical and physiological

fitness. Conversely, increases in physical activity may increase absolute or sustained force or power. Adequate levels of muscular power and endurance enable human beings to perform the activities of daily living throughout their varied life spans.

Within a motor unit, properties of fibers are more homogenous than throughout whole muscles. The fibers within a given motor unit may be classified as slow, fast fatigue resistant, or fast fatiguable. Muscle fibers may also be classified on the basis of myofibrillar ATPase activity (Type I, Type IIA, Type IIB, Type IIC) or the activities of both the myofibrillar ATPase and oxidative enzymes (slow-oxidative, fast-oxidative-glycolytic, and fast-glycolytic). The numbers and sizes of the different types of motor units in a given muscle determine functional capability. Recruitment of motor units occurs on the basis of size, from small, slow units for low intensity tasks, through the additional recruitment of fast fatigue resistant units for moderate intensity tasks, to fast fatiguable units for high intensity tasks. The interaction of the recruitment pattern and the habitual intensity of daily physical activity play a key role in motor unit adaptation and consequently the characteristics of the muscle fibers.

Physical activities involve various combinations of shortening, isometric, and lengthening contractions. Shortening contractions generate the power for movements of the organism or of external objects, and are energetically demanding. Measurements of work performed or power output provide the best estimates of the intensity of physical activity. The response can only be compared in terms of relative intensities of the maximum power during a single contraction.

Fatigue is defined as a loss in the development of force and/or velocity, that results from physical activity, and is reversible by rest. Fatigue is induced by accumulation of the products of ATP hydrolysis, including inorganic phosphate and hydrogen ions, which can potentially impair excitation-contraction coupling in the muscle. In longterm physical activity, a depletion of muscle glycogen stores may impair the ability of the muscle to develop force. Depending on the intensity and duration of the physical activity, full recovery occurs within minutes or hours. Decreases in force development that persist for more than 24 hours after physical activity are due to contraction-induced injury.

Training modifies the morphological, metabolic and molecular properties of muscle, altering the functional attributes of fibers in specific motor units. Adaptations for strength and endurance may occur independently, although training programs may produce increases in both attributes.

Bed-rest, immobilization, and weightlessness reduce recruitment and/or loading. Each model has differing effects. Immobilization and weightlessness result in a decrease in muscle mass and in the cross-sectional area of single fibers. Maintenance of a given level of physiological fitness requires a certain intensity, duration, and frequency of physical activity. Following a period of sustained increase or decrease in physical activity, adaptations may be reversed. During detraining, muscle fiber changes regress toward pretraining values, but some adaptations are sustained for considerable periods of time. The decrease in absolute force results from both the decrease in muscle cross-sectional area, and reduction in force developed per unit area.

During the early stages of strength training, maximum power can increase as a result of neurophysiological adaptations despite the absence of morphological or biochemical changes. Heavy-resistance strength training subsequently results in an increase in muscle cross-sectional area in all three fiber types. In addition, the proportion of Type IIA fiber subtypes is altered. Following ablation of synergistic muscles, the myosin isoform expression shifts from the fast toward slow-type. Peptide mapping suggests that a true transformation of myosin occurs in the hypertrophied fibers.

Endurance training increases the capacity of muscles to sustain force and power. The primary adaptations to prolonged physical activity are metabolic, hormonal, and cardiovascular changes that enhance the ability to oxidize all fuels including fatty acids during prolonged physical activity, to conserve carbohydrates (particularly muscle glycogen concentration), and to attenuate metabolic acidosis. If the intensity and duration of the endurance training program is sufficient, mitochondrial capacity increases in all fiber types. Although endurance training reduces blood flow during submaximal exercise, higher blood flows to the contracting muscles are observed during exercise at high intensities. Endurance training programs do not appear to induce any substantial changes in the major fiber types. For most individuals of all ages, increased physical activity and the associated improvements in strength, power, and endurance has the potential to improve the intensity and diversity of daily activities that can be performed without fatigue or the possibility of injury. This increase in capacity for the activities of daily living improves quality of life.

IMPORTANT RESEARCH TOPICS

77. To determine the mechanism responsible for fatigue during different intensities of physical activity.
78. To establish the interrelationships among the measurements made on skeletal muscle in vitro, in situ, and in vivo and the validity of extrapolating from observations on single permeabilized fibers to fibers in vivo.
79. To determine the relative role of the type of muscle progenitor cells and the subsequent environmental factors that ultimately result in diverse populations of muscle cells.
80. To determine the functional significance of the diversity of protein isoforms of muscle throughout the life span.
81. To establish the biomechanical behaviors of synergistic muscles during varied programs of exercise.
82. To establish the basis for age-related deficits that occur in skeletal muscles.
83. To determine the effects of training programs on the properties of skeletal muscle fibers.
84. To establish the significance of specific muscle adaptations in modifying hormonal, electrolyte, metabolic, and cardiovascular capacities.
85. To determine mechanisms underlying susceptibility to, and recovery from, the injury to skeletal muscle induced by various forms of exercise.
86. To develop programs of regular muscular activity that are affordable, safe, and acceptable to large numbers of sedentary people.

Physical Activity and Adipose Tissue

Adipose tissue is the most important organ for lipid storage. During prolonged exercise, the fuel mixture oxidized by the skeletal muscle varies, depending upon the intensity and the duration of exercise, but lipid mobilized from adipose tissue contributes significantly to the energy supply.

Endurance training can induce net lipid mobilization from adipose tissue, eventually leading to a reduction in adipose tissue mass if the increased mobilization is not fully compensated by mechanisms increasing lipid storage. To reduce adipose tissue mass, an exercise program without dietary restriction must generate a substantial energy expenditure, and the minimal prescription commonly recommended for improving cardiorespiratory fitness is often insufficient. Under these circumstances, dietary interventions generally produce a greater energy deficit, and thus, faster rates of decrease in body mass than exercise training alone. Weight loss induced by endurance training is, however, associated with a better preservation of fat free mass than hypocaloric diets. With endurance training, men generally show a greater reduction in body fat than women. Metabolic improvements associated with the reduction of adipose tissue mass include changes of carbohydrate and lipid metabolism that may reduce the risk of developing diabetes and cardiovascular disease.

The regulation of adipose tissue mass depends upon several metabolic processes, including lipolysis, and reesterification and storage through the hydrolysis of circulating triglycerides by the enzyme lipoprotein lipase. In lean subjects, endurance training increases the lipolytic response of adipose cells to catecholamines. Adipose tissue lipoprotein lipase is also increased, which contributes to the replenishment of adipose tissue lipid stores between exercise sessions. Much less information is available regarding obese subjects. Gender and site-specific differences in the response of adipose tissue lipolysis to catecholamines have been reported, this variation being partly attributed to alterations in the ratio of alpha (inhibitory) to beta (stimulatory) adrenergic receptors. The relative role of these factors in the response of adipose tissue lipolysis to exercise training has not been established. Gender differences in the acute response of abdominal and femoral adipose cell lipolysis to endurance exercise have been reported. Gluteal adipose cell lipolytic response to catecholamines is acutely increased following endurance exercise in men but not in women. These results may explain the apparently greater ability of men to lose gluteal fat in response to training. The response of adipose tissue lipoprotein lipase to insulin is increased in obese patients after weight loss. No information is currently available on the effects of endurance training on the regulation of adipose tissue lipoprotein lipase activity by insulin in humans.

Processes other than lipoprotein lipase activity must be involved in lipid accretion in adipose cells, as a normal adipose tissue mass has been reported in individuals with no lipoprotein lipase activity. Insulin-stimulated glucose transport is increased in adipose cells after training, which may contribute to the replenishment of adipose tissue lipids after exercise.

Plainly, human adipose tissue metabolism can adapt to endurance training. Endurance training that generates a large energy expenditure can reduce adipose tissue fat mass. Upper body fat is more readily mobilized than lower body fat during training. Endurance training may reduce the quantity of atherogenic visceral adipose tissue, especially when initial levels are high. Factors influencing the response of visceral adipose tissue to training include gender and age, as well as the initial stores of total body and abdominal visceral fat. The abdominal adipose depot appears to be more readily mobilized than peripheral depots. Reductions in adipose tissue mass are a consequence of decreases in average adipose cell size, but there is no change in fat cell number.

IMPORTANT RESEARCH TOPICS

87. Which mechanisms are responsible for the apparently greater loss of body fat in response to endurance training in men than in women?
88. What are the gender and site-specific differences in the effects of endurance training on adipose tissue metabolism?
89. What are the effects of endurance training on adipose tissue metabolism in various age groups and under various hormonal conditions (menopause, hormone replacement)?
90. Is there any relationship between the phase of the menstrual cycle, reproductive status, and the acute response of adipose tissue metabolism to exercise?
91. Are there differences between obese and lean individuals in the effects of endurance training on the metabolism of adipose cells obtained from various depots?
92. How does insulin regulate lipoprotein lipase activity in adipose tissue and its acute and chronic response to endurance exercise?
93. What are the mechanisms responsible for the genetic variation in the response of adipose tissue metabolism to endurance training?

Physical Activity and Connective Tissue

Connective tissue is the most abundant tissue type of the human body. Among the various forms of connective tissue, the dense fibrous elements (bone, ligament, tendon, and cartilage) have been the most studied under conditions of habitual exercise. However, increasing research interest has recently been directed toward exercise-induced adaptations of connective tissue in cardiac and skeletal muscle. The fibrillar collagen network in bones, ligaments, tendons and cartilage is more compact than the collagen domain in skeletal muscle. Composition, micro-architecture, cell type, and metabolism vary among the forms of connective tissue. It has been suggested that the adaptation of morphological, biochemical, and biomechanical properties to exercise is driven primarily by physical forces. The biomechanical aspects of locomotion (torsion, compression, and tension) translate into changes in mechanical stresses that present local elements of skeletal muscle, bone, ligament, cartilage, and tendon with a unique load history. This load history alters connective tissue metabolism and structure, leading to unique tissue adaptations. The biomechanical parameters of exercise characterize the types of activity that produce particular adaptations. Therefore, a specific characterization of the exercise undertaken is essential in determining the characteristics of connective tissue adaptation.

Unfortunately, there is a dearth of information characterizing and quantifying the in vivo load histories of the connective tissues in the various body segments. Few have been successful in measuring in vivo tissue loads and/or strains during exercise in human and animal models. Therefore, the approach of scientists has been focused primarily on tissue adaptations to exercise with the assumption that they are the result of physical challenges. This approach is partly valid, because connective tissue structural adaptation does not always follow Wolff's Law which asserts that change in connective tissue mass is directly proportional to the magnitude of the applied force. In addition, the level of tissue organization is a function of the direction of the applied force. However, the exercise stimulus involves not only biomechanical criteria, but also alterations of endocrine profile. Connective tissue anabolism and catabolism (turnover) are modified by exercise. Studies have documented exercise-induced endocrine changes which have the potential to alter connective tissue turnover and structure.

Exercise stimulates the metabolism of connective tissues. Nonetheless, not all studies support the hypothesis that exercise alone enhances connective tissue strength and organization. Other factors such as age, diet, endocrine status, and environment can enhance or reduce the effects of exercise.

Increases in the circulating metabolites of connective tissue structural proteins are seen in marathon runners, indicating an increase of tissue turnover. Biopsy data in both humans and animals verify that exercise increases the secretion and resorption of extracellular matrix proteins. The changes in concentration of these metabolites vary with time, indicating the temporal basis of connective tissue responses to exercise. Tissue studies support the hypothesis that exercise adaptation is multiphasic. For example, exercise "up-regulates" the synthesis and secretion of collagen, but there is a "down-regulation" in the formation of stable collagen crosslinks (a marker of maturation). However, at some point in time, a steady-state of adaptation is achieved and maturation is enhanced. Collagen has a long half-life in many of the dense fibrous connective tissues (110 days in tendon) and continues to be modified throughout the life of the protein. It is uncertain whether exercise alters the half-life of mature collagen.

Some preliminary evidence suggests that strenuous exercise increases the degradation of mature collagen. This would imply that an initial phase of connective tissue adaptation involves the resorption of mature collagen and its replacement by "younger" protein with fewer stable crosslinks. Other evidence shows that tissues of strenuously exercised rats have relatively more (percent of total) connective tissue mass, with fewer stable collagen crosslinks, resulting in a lower maximum stress and elastic modulus. However, the structural and material properties of connective tissues improve as the duration of training is increased. Most studies have reported results at a single point in time. This may partly account for the lack of consensus regarding connective tissue adaptations to exercise.

IMPORTANT RESEARCH TOPICS

94. The exercise dose-response should be evaluated for connective tissue structure and organization over various time periods.

95. Quantitative in vivo force-displacement data should be collected during locomotion.
96. An in-depth examination of connective tissue adaptations should be made in populations of differing age, sex, endocrine status, diet, and disease state in various environments.
97. Biomarkers of connective tissue metabolism in various body fluids should be validated to allow measurements during training.
98. Changes in such biomarkers should be correlated with the short- and long-term effects of exercise on the musculoskeletal system.
99. A non-invasive technology should be developed to assess connective tissue responses to exercise.
100. Studies should determine whether acute exercise causes degradation of mature collagen.

Physical Activity and Digestive Processes

Gastrointestinal symptoms are a common source of disability. The interaction between physical activity and the digestive processes is complex. We lack primary knowledge of much of the basic gastrointestinal physiology associated with exercise. Investigative techniques are hampered by artifacts from body motion, variations in study populations, and differing exercise test protocols. However, significant acute gastrointestinal problems such as nausea, vomiting, diarrhea, and gastrointestinal bleeding are associated with exercise. There are few studies of adaptations of the gastrointestinal system to chronic exercise, or the influence of exercise on gastrointestinal disease.

Surveys suggest that endurance runners have a relatively high frequency of digestive complaints, particularly nausea and diarrhea. Other symptoms include: a frequent urge to defecate or actual defecation with exercise, abdominal cramps, a loss of appetite, heartburn, chest pain, belching, and rarely, rectal bleeding. These complaints, while usually not severe, are troublesome and may impair exercise performance.

Studies examining the effects of exercise on gastroesophageal reflux show it to be potentiated by exercise, particularly when running postprandially. Acid exposure can be controlled by histamine receptor blockade. Esophageal motility changes with exercise. Low- and moderate-intensity exercise accelerates gastric emptying of liquid, while high intensity exercise delays it. Changes in the gastric emptying of solids appear similar, but data are more limited. Scanty data suggest only minor changes in gastric acid secretion with exercise. Changes in small intestinal motility and absorption with moderate exercise are also small, and of uncertain clinical significance. Colonic transit is unchanged or accelerated by both moderate exercise and aerobic training. The etiology of exercise-associated gastrointestinal motility changes may include alterations in visceral blood flow, neurohormonal axis, abdominal pressure and position, trauma, and medications.

The gastrointestinal hemorrhage that is associated with exercise may present as occult, asymptomatic bleeding, but less commonly and potentially more seriously, it may also manifest itself as acute bleeding from gastritis or colitis. Possible etiologies include ischemic damage, trauma, the effects of chronic medications including aspirin and non-steroidal anti-inflammatory drugs, and underlying pre-existent disease. Small randomized clinical trials suggest that cimetidine may be an effective therapy in selected cases of gastrointestinal bleeding.

Liver-associated enzyme activities may be abnormal transiently following strenuous exercise, but such changes rarely reflect significant hepatic disease or damage. Exercise acutely reduces hepatic blood flow. Aerobic training may enhance hepatic synthetic function as manifested by increased rates of aminopyrine and antipyrine metabolism.

IMPORTANT RESEARCH TOPICS

101. There is a pressing need to improve investigative techniques for evaluation of gastrointestinal physiology during exercise.
102. The etiology of exercise-induced gastrointestinal symptoms such as nausea, vomiting, diarrhea, and abdominal pain, and its relation to recognized gastrointestinal physiologic changes, needs to be established.
103. The physiological mechanisms responsible for exercise-related alterations in gastric emptying require clarification.

104. The pathophysiology and therapy of exercise-associated gastrointestinal hemorrhage remains unknown, and further work is required to elucidate it.
105. The interaction of exercise with diseases of the gastrointestinal system remains to be explored.
106. Liver, biliary system, and pancreatic function should be evaluated during exercise in both health and disease.

Physical Activity and Carbohydrate Metabolism

Many exergonic processes occur in skeletal muscle cells, but during contraction the hydrolysis of ATP becomes dominant. Whereas the phosphorylation of ADP is immediately accomplished by creatine phosphate and creatine phosphotransferase, sustained contractions require the participation of glycolysis and oxidative phosphorylation to maintain the mitochondrial-chemiosmotic gradient, and thus, the cellular ATP-ADP ratio. Muscle glycogenolysis and glycolysis provide the energy for short bursts of activity.

In sustained aerobic activity, carbohydrate utilization through glycolysis is again the main source of reducing equivalents for mitochondrial respiration during moderate- or high-intensity exercise. The availability of carbohydrates in the form of exogenous (blood) glucose is required for optimal cardiac function both in isolated working rabbit hearts, as well as in the intact beating human heart. The transition of rest to exercise is marked by increased utilization of most fuel sources, with the greatest relative gain in the utilization of muscle carbohydrate (glycogen). Muscle glycogen depletion is associated with fatigue. Thus, carbohydrate availability is required to support the energy needs of exercise of moderate or greater intensity.

Whereas the rate of mitochondrial respiration is tightly coupled to the energetics of muscle contraction, the coupling between glycolytic flux and mitochondrial requirements for oxidizable substrates is looser. Muscle contraction induces both increased glucose uptake and glycogenolysis. Additionally, epinephrine (Beta 2-adrenergic stimulation) can accelerate the rate of glycogenolysis in resting as well as contracting muscle. Thus, resting and contracting muscle both show a net release of lactate, especially at the onset of exercise or under the influence of epinephrine.

Lactate released from contracting skeletal muscle and other storage sites (e.g., inactive muscle, adipose, liver) may serve as a fuel source at cellular sites with a high rate of respiration (e.g., heart, lung, and red skeletal muscle). In post-absorptive human beings, exercising at approximately 50% of $\dot{V}O_2$max, the utilization of blood lactate approximates that of glucose. At higher relative power outputs, or with the imposition of added stress such as the hypobaric hypoxia of altitude, the utilization of blood lactate can even exceed that of glucose.

In the postprandial state, hepatic glucose production may be supported by glycogenolysis and gluconeogenesis. During prolonged exercise in the post-absorptive state, gluconeogenesis from lactate (i.e., the Cori Cycle) becomes essential for the maintenance of hepatic glucose production and thus blood glucose homeostasis. Under the latter circumstances, gluconeogenic or Beta 2-adrenergic blockade results in a fall of hepatic glucose production, hypoglycemia, and fatigue.

Resting muscle utilizes only a relatively small proportion of hepatic glucose production. During moderate- to high-intensity exercise, the significant increase in metabolic rate and overall carbohydrate utilization of the contracting muscle require a redistribution of glucose flux. However, the increase of hepatic glucose production during exercise still provides only a small fraction of the carbohydrate utilized by the contracting muscle at the onset of exercise or during moderate- to high-intensity exercise. The majority of the carbohydrates required by the contracting muscle is derived from intramuscular glycogen stores.

Synthesis accompanies the degradation of skeletal muscle glycogen during exercise. Studies utilizing infusion of ^{3}H-glucose and ^{14}C-lactate into laboratory animals demonstrate the incorporation of glucose into muscle and liver glycogen pools, including tissues where net glycogenolysis is occurring.

The increased lipid oxidation capacity of trained muscle spares glycogen during exercise, and the increased glucose uptake capacity may promote glycogen storage during recovery from exercise. A training-induced increased mass of mitochondrial reticulum allows a greater oxidation of both carbohydrate and lipid in high-intensity exercise; it also permits increased lipid utilization, and glycogen sparing during moderate-intensity exercise.

Endogenous carbohydrate fuel sources are of primary importance in sustaining physical activities ranging from short bursts to prolonged exercise. Complex cell-to-cell and tissue-to-tissue interactions are involved in the supply of glucose and lactate as energy sources for muscle contraction during exercise. Local contraction-induced events as well as the sympathetic-adrenal system appear extremely important in controlling the exchange of carbohydrate energy forms during exercise.

IMPORTANT RESEARCH TOPICS

107. What are the pathways of hexose disposal during rest, exercise, and recovery?
108. What are the regulating factors which allow whole-body muscle glycogen stores to be mobilized during sustained exercise?
109. How is the fuel selection of exercising muscle regulated?
110. Which healthful dietary habits can be encouraged to improve exercise tolerance in both the general population and athletes?
111. What are the mechanisms which allow substrates to interact to supply fuels during exercise? For instance, how effective is increased muscle glucose uptake and supporting glycogenolysis during exercise?

Physical Activity, Lipid and Lipoprotein Metabolism, and Lipid Transport

The class of compounds described as lipids is quite diverse. However, only free fatty acids which are stored in their ester form (triacylglycerols or triglycerides) are important as a metabolic fuel. To utilize lipids as fuel, the muscle must take up, activate, and translocate free fatty acids into mitochondria, supplying acetyl coenzyme A to the citric acid cycle. Sources of free fatty acids for oxidation include: (a) circulating free fatty acids, which are mobilized from adipose tissue following hydrolysis of stored triglycerides by hormone-sensitive lipase; (b) circulating lipoprotein triglycerides, which are hydrolyzed on the surface of the muscle capillary endothelium by lipoprotein lipase, the activity of which is relatively high in cardiac and oxidative skeletal muscle fibers; and (c) intramuscular triglycerides, which are more abundant in oxidative muscle fibers. Utilization of free fatty acids during exercise depends on the intensity of activity, the subject's state of training and the diet.

In acute response to physical activity, fat is oxidized in progressively increasing amounts as the total energy expenditure increases, so that lipids may cover up to 90% of oxidative metabolism in prolonged bouts of exercise (greater than one hour) at moderate-intensity ($< 50\%$ $\dot{V}O_2$max). As the intensity of exercise increases ($> 70\%$ $\dot{V}O_2$max), fat is used in decreasing amounts, and glycogen becomes the predominant energy source.

With the onset of exercise, an initial fall in plasma free fatty acids concentration, arising from an increased uptake by the working muscle, is followed by increased plasma free fatty acid levels. This is due to liberation of free fatty acids from adipose tissue as lipolysis is stimulated by hormone-sensitive lipase activity in response to increased sympathoadrenal activity and decreased insulin levels. A major fraction of the free fatty acids liberated is reesterified within the adipocyte. Free fatty acids, which are released into the blood stream, are bound to the protein albumin and are transported to the working muscle. For any given individual and exercise intensity, there is a close relationship between the arterial free fatty acid concentration and the amount of free fatty acids taken up and oxidized in muscles. However, several lines of evidence suggest that hydrolysis of circulating lipoprotein triglycerides and intramuscular triglycerides contribute to the provision of free fatty acids for exercising muscles. The latter sources may be of greater importance following endurance training or consumption of a high-fat diet.

Endurance training increases the capability for fat oxidation. The absolute mass of the skeletal muscle mitochondria increases with training, resulting in increased concentrations of enzymes for the citric acid cycle, fatty acid and ketone body oxidation, and the electron transfer system. There is a greater reliance on fat as a source of energy during submaximal exercise at the same absolute work rate in trained individuals. Endurance training results in an increased lipolytic responsiveness to Beta-adrenergic stimulation, concomitant with lower plasma catecholamine concentrations. Training increases the activity of both skeletal muscle and adipose tissue lipoprotein lipase, thereby facilitating the use of circulating triglycerides as a fuel source in trained muscles and promoting the clearance of circulating triglycerides even at rest.

Active men and women generally exhibit decreased plasma concentrations of triglycerides and increased levels of high-density lipoprotein cholesterol in comparison with sedentary individuals, suggesting that their risk of heart disease is reduced. Randomized, controlled clinical trials of at least 12 weeks duration show that sedentary men who adopt a program of regular aerobic exercise reduce plasma triglycerides and increase high-density lipoprotein cholesterol. There are fewer similar studies in women that have yielded less consistent results; however, these also generally show decreases in plasma triglycerides. Loss of body fat generally accompanies increases in aerobic exercise when the intake of food energy is unchanged or reduced, and is occasionally seen even if food intake is increased, if the training is long and hard enough. Fat loss may bring about changes in lipoproteins, even in the absence of exercise, but several lines of evidence suggest that exercise training affects lipoproteins independently of fat loss. Increased skeletal muscle lipoprotein lipase activity, for instance, contributes to lipoprotein metabolism. In single-leg training studies, lipoprotein triglycerides is lower and high-density lipoprotein cholesterol is higher in blood draining the trained leg compared to arterial blood, but no such differences are seen in the untrained leg. Exercise training can result in a reduction in total and abdominal fat which may contribute further to long-term improvements in lipoprotein metabolism. Additionally, changes in diet composition (relative quantity of fat and carbohydrate) can significantly modify the effects of training on lipoproteins. It remains to be determined whether sex differences are important in the effects of training on lipid and lipoprotein metabolism.

IMPORTANT RESEARCH TOPICS

112. How is fuel selection regulated during exercise?
113. What variables influence the sources of fatty acid, which are utilized as fuels, during exercise?
114. What is the best nutritional plan to optimize fat utilization during exercise without impairing performance?
115. Is there an optimal work intensity, frequency, and duration that maximizes fat utilization in most individuals bringing about the greatest benefits in weight regulation and weight-related problems, such as lipoprotein disorders and diabetes?

116. Which diet and exercise programs would increase the utilization of centrally-deposited fat?
117. Are there sex differences in the influence of exercise upon lipid and lipoprotein metabolism, and do these differ across the life cycle?

Physical Activity, Protein, and Amino Acid Metabolism

Exercise is associated with an increased catabolism of protein and amino acids. This is shown by an increased production of urea (with an increased nitrogen excretion in sweat and urine) and increased amino acid oxidation (as shown by production of labelled CO_2 from ^{13}C and ^{14}C carboxyl-labelled leucine and $^{15}NH_3$ from ^{15}N glycine). The net negative nitrogen balance may be masked, unless precautions are taken to account for losses in sweat, the delayed pattern of urinary nitrogen excretion, and the difficulty of observing small changes in the large body urea pool. However, the use of stable-isotope tracers to follow urea production rate and the transfer of label from amino acids to labelled urea suggests that urea production increases less than would be expected from other measures (e.g., leucine oxidation and the amount of amino acid delivered to the liver). The contradiction may be resolved if, as seems likely, exercise causes the liver to increase the production of acute phase proteins (such as fibrinogen or fibronectin). These substances are relatively branched-chain amino acid depleted compared to tissue protein, which is the likely source of the branched-chain amino acids oxidized in exercise.

The amount of amino acids in the free tissue and blood amino acid pool is increased during short-term exercise. This increase is almost certainly due to a fall in the ratio of whole body protein synthesis to breakdown. During high-intensity short-term exercise, ammonia production increases markedly, probably as a result of the action of adenosine deaminase at the expense of AMP, without replenishment of AMP from amino acids. Alanine production increases in this type of exercise to the extent that pyruvate is made available by glycolysis; this may help to limit acidosis. In longer-term exercise, some amino acid pools are diminished markedly. For example, muscle glutamate and blood branched-chain amino acids fall, probably due to an increased rate of transamination of branched-chain amino acids; whereas the production of alanine, aspartate, glutamine and ammonia rises. The exact source of carbon for the amino acids exported from muscle in this type of exercise remains unclear; muscle protein, glycogen and glucose are all possible precursors. The proportion of each is unknown, and may vary according to substrate availability.

During exercise, branched-chain amino acid oxidation is increased; this is due to an increased delivery (branched-chain amino acid transporters have a high capacity, but a low affinity), an increased net muscle breakdown, and an increase in the proportion of the branched chain ketoacid dehydrogenase that is in the active form. Activation of the dehydrogenase is closely correlated with metabolic state and probably also with the intensity and duration of exercise. It is inversely correlated with pre-existing glycogen stores, so that amino acid oxidation would be minimized under conditions of high glycogen availability.

Amino acid oxidation contributes a small fraction of energy needs compared with that derived from other fuels. It may nevertheless be important in sparing other sources of glucose and in providing a source of new carbon for gluconeogenesis. There is growing evidence that branched-chain amino acid oxidation is incomplete and branched-chain hydroxyacids are released from muscle to gluconeogenic tissues. The exercise-induced efflux of alanine and glutamine from muscle is taken up by the splanchnic bed, thus enabling the cycling of nitrogen from the periphery to the viscera with potential benefits for pH regulation and gluconeogenesis.

There is an acute decrease of protein synthesis in contracting muscle during exercise. Possible causes include a fall in ATP:ADP and in ribosome aggregation. There is conflicting evidence concerning muscle protein breakdown during exercise. Some workers claim that it is depressed and others that it is elevated. Part of the confusion may be due to the heterogeneity of the protein pool and the many proteolytic processes involved (e.g., ATP-dependent and independent processes would react differently). There may also be a time-dependent phenomenon, with muscle breakdown being depressed during exercise but elevated afterwards.

There is no doubt that muscle protein synthesis can rise markedly after exercise. The changes are so large they suggest that a remodeling-associated increase in breakdown must also occur, since the total protein mass increases relatively slowly. In young healthy men, there is no evidence that growth hormone supplements increase muscle protein accretion, although growth hormone may help rehabilitation after injury and in the maintenance of muscle mass in elderly men. Immobilization results in wasting because of a fall in muscle protein synthesis. This can be minimized by early remobilization or electrical stimulation.

The influence of large muscle exercise on dietary protein requirements is equivocal. During aerobic exercise, the increased utilization of some essential amino acids (e.g., the branched-chain amino acids) suggests that dietary protein requirements might be increased. This might be important for people living on a low protein diet (e.g., vegetarians or people of the developing world), or for any individual maintaining activity on an energy-reduced slimming diet. Nevertheless, there is no good evidence of any such change in requirements. Even if there were, because of the protein dense nature of the diet of most people in the developed world, satisfaction of energy requirements would inevitably satisfy protein needs for omnivores.

During an increase in training, individuals may show an adaptive increase in protein accretion. There is little evidence to suggest that once a plateau of fitness is reached, protein turnover (expressed per unit of lean body mass) is elevated by habitual exercise. Habitual exercise probably has a beneficial effect in maintaining muscle mass (and possibly protein turnover) in the elderly.

IMPORTANT RESEARCH TOPICS

118. Why is it so difficult to see the expected changes in urea turnover in relation to branched-chain amino acid oxidation? Can synthesis of acute phase proteins during or after exercise explain the "mopping up" of amino acids released from body protein?

119. Are the partial oxidation products of valine and isoleucine (their hydroxy acid analogues) an important source of carbon for gluconeogenesis?

120. Do amino acid and protein metabolism have roles in acid-base homeostasis during and after exercise?

121. What changes in turnover of specific proteins occur in muscle during and after exercise and what are the mechanisms?

122. Does exercise increase protein requirements and is this important for people on low-protein diets?

123. What interplay exists between growth or aging and exercise-induced changes in protein and amino acid metabolism?
124. What influence does a manipulation of the carbohydrate and protein content of the diet have on protein metabolism during exercise and training?

Physical Activity, Fitness, Immune Function, and Glutamine

There is limited evidence that some forms of low-intensity exercise may be beneficial to the immune system, whereas high intensity and long duration exercise may be detrimental to the immune system. There is a nutritional link between muscle and the immune system, which might in part explain the effects of exercise on immune function.

Lymphocytes and macrophages play a quantitatively important role in the immune response, undergoing increased rates of production, recruitment, and activity. It has generally been thought that lymphocytes and macrophages obtain most of their energy by metabolism of glucose, and that resting lymphocytes, which have not been subjected to an immune response, are metabolically and nutritionally quiescent. This is not so. Glutamine is an extremely important fuel for both macrophages and lymphocytes: the rate of glutamine utilization is similar to or even greater than that of glucose. However, neutrophils do not appear to use glutamine at such a high rate. A high rate of glutamine utilization, but only partial oxidation, is characteristic of other cells (enterocytes, thymocytes, colonocytes, fibroblasts, and possibly endothelial cells). A hypothesis has been put forward which suggests that a high rate of glutamine utilization provides optimal conditions to regulate the use of the intermediates of the glutamine utilization pathway for synthesis of such compounds as purine and pyrimidine nucleotides for DNA and RNA synthesis essential for proliferation of cells. A decrease in the rate of glutamine utilization by lymphocytes would thus be expected to decrease the rate of cell proliferation. This has been shown to be the case in cultures of rat and human lymphocytes.

The importance of a high rate of glutamine utilization by these cells may be to permit a rapid immune response. The overall rate of glutamine utilization may be very high, since there are many lymphocytes in the body (approximately 1500 g in humans). This raises the important questions of the source and availability of this glutamine.

Glutamine is made available in the lumen of the intestine from the digestion of protein. However, the absorptive cells of the small intestine probably utilize almost all that is absorbed from a normal diet unsupplemented with glutamine. A major tissue involved in endogenous glutamine production is skeletal muscle: it contains a high concentration of glutamine, it has the enzymic capacity to synthesize glutamine, and it is known to release glutamine into the bloodstream at a varying rate.

The key process in the control of the rate of glutamine release by muscle is the glutamine transporter that carries glutamine across the plasma membrane. The rate of this process may be influenced by a number of hormones. Consequently, the process of glutamine synthesis may not be important to the acute control of glutamine release by muscle. Subsequently, this would impact on the plasma concentration of free glutamine.

Muscle can then be considered an important tissue source for providing substrate to the immune system. Failure of muscle to provide enough glutamine could result in impaired immune function. Therefore, an important question is what happens to the plasma glutamine levels after exercise?

Preliminary investigation in human subjects suggests that changes in the level of plasma glutamine during exercise varies with the nature of the exercise task. For example, the plasma glutamine concentration is decreased after a 42-km marathon but increased after sprints. Similarly, in the overtrained state, the plasma glutamine concentration is significantly lower in overtrained athletes compared with that in optimally trained athletes. The concentrations of alanine and branched-chain amino acids are similar in the plasma of trained and overtrained athletes. These changes are consistent with the hypothesis that a variation in the rate of glutamine release by muscle could influence the ability of the immune system to respond to an immune challenge.

IMPORTANT RESEARCH TOPICS

125. What happens to the plasma glutamine level when overtrained athletes engage in acute exercise?
126. What is the effect of different intensities and durations of exercise on arteriovenous differences in glutamine concentration for legs or arms in humans?

127. Do lymphocytes in vivo utilize glutamine at rates consistent with those predicted from in vitro experiments?
128. Will the provision of glutamine or glutamine-containing peptides during and/or after strenuous bouts of exercise decrease the risk of upper respiratory tract infections associated with such activity?
129. What is the effect of various training regimes on the plasma glutamine level?
130. Would previous exercise training facilitate glutamine release from muscle after undergoing surgery, thus improving the rate of recovery of the patient?

Physical Activity and Iron Metabolism

The belief that regular physical activity causes a specific anemia, the so-called "sports anemia," is entrenched in the scientific literature. However, the criteria for diagnosing such an anemia are inadequate. Thus, the incidence of the condition and its etiology are not clearly established.

The increased frequency of abnormalities in biochemical measures of iron status in the physically active individual, including low serum ferritin concentrations (8 to 22% in males; 9 to 82% in females), reduced hemoglobin concentrations (9 to 60%) and absence of stainable bone marrow stores, suggest that regular physical activity can impair whole-body iron metabolism. Factors that might explain these findings include: iron deficiency, increased rates of hemolysis, a dilutional effect, or activation of an acute phase response.

Conventional biochemical criteria for the diagnosis of iron-deficiency anemia include a blood hemoglobin concentration lower than 140 g/l in males and 120 g/l in females and one or both of the following: < 12 mg/l serum ferritin concentration, and < 18% transferrin saturation. When these stringent criteria are used to diagnose iron-deficiency anemia in the physically-active, the prevalence of iron deficiency ranges between 0 to 4% in both men and women. The prevalence in active women is not different from that of sedentary females but the prevalence in active males is higher than in the general population.

Factors that may explain changes in measures of iron status in the physically active include: a low intake of heme-iron, especially in vegetarian athletes; increased iron losses in sweat, urine, and feces (although these losses are typically small in normal subjects); impaired gastrointestinal iron absorption, and a disproportionate increase in blood volume relative to the increase in red cell mass causing a dilutional "pseudo anemia." These changes are not part of an acute phase response.

Iron therapy improves the exercise capacity of subjects with proven iron deficiency. A number of studies show that treatment of subjects with either low serum ferritin concentrations or reduced hemoglobin concentrations do not influence laboratory measures of maximal exercise performance.

IMPORTANT RESEARCH TOPICS

131. There is a need to establish adequate criteria for the assessment of hematological status in physically active individuals. The prevalence and etiology of iron deficiency and iron deficiency anemia need to be determined on the basis of these criteria.
132. There is a need to study the possibility that whole-body iron kinetics is substantially altered in the physically active person. In particular, there is a need to determine the cause of the low serum ferritin concentrations in the physically active.
133. There is a need to study whether iron therapy enhances prolonged submaximal exercise performance in individuals with low serum ferritin concentrations without anemia, or vice versa.

Physical Activity, Fibrinolysis, and Platelet Aggregability

Blood coagulation, fibrinolysis and platelet aggregation are intimately involved with early as well as advanced stages of atherosclerosis. The majority of published data relating physical activity with coagulation, fibrinolysis, and platelet function are restricted to young healthy subjects who have been exposed to a single bout of physical exercise. Measurements suggest that heavy exercise transiently increases in vitro blood coagulation, whereas moderate intensity effort is sufficient to activate fibrinolysis. Acute effects on platelet aggregability remain to be elucidated.

Available data suggest decreased plasma fibrinogen concentration, increased fibrinolytic and diminished antifibrinolytic activity after intensive exercise training in clinically healthy older men. In addition, limited data in middle-aged, overweight, mildly hypertensive men suggest that regular moderate-intensity exercise training inhibits platelet aggregability.

IMPORTANT RESEARCH TOPICS

---

134. Does physical activity have a dose-response related influence on blood coagulation, fibrinolysis, and platelet function?
135. What are the temporal relationships of any effects of physical activity on blood coagulation, fibrinolysis, and platelet function?
136. Do drugs, diet and physical activity have interactive effects on blood coagulation, fibrinolysis, and platelet aggregability?
137. Does physical activity influence the thrombotic mechanisms involved in atherosclerosis?

Physical Activity and Free Radicals

Oxygen-free radicals are essential in certain physiologic reactions, but can be potentially harmful, and contribute to several human diseases. If oxygen-free radicals accumulate unduly in cells, they can damage DNA, protein, and lipids. The body defends against oxygen-free radicals by means of scavenger enzymes, metal-binding proteins, and "antioxidants" such as vitamins E, C, and beta carotene.

Because oxygen-free radicals form during normal aerobic metabolism, they may be harmful to tissues, especially those with high rates of oxygen utilization or those subject to ischemia/reperfusion during exercise. Consequently, researchers are exploring the possible roles of oxygen-free radicals in physical activity, health, and disease.

Clinical research is hampered because assays for oxygen-free radicals are indirect and lack standardization. The most commonly used methods gauge either consumption of "antioxidants" (for instance, changes in blood concentrations of reduced glutathione) or the production of "oxidant damage," as measured by lipid peroxidation products in breath (pentane) or serum (thiobarbituric, acid-reactive substances).

The few studies of oxygen-free radicals in exercisers show these trends:

• Vigorous exercise tends to increase breath pentane production and serum thiobarbituric, acid-reactive substance concentration, and/or lower erythrocyte reduced glutathione concentration.

• Increments in serum concentrations of muscle enzymes (e.g., creatine kinase) tend to parallel increments in serum thiobarbituric, acid-reactive substances in exercisers with a known eccentric or tissue-damaging component.

• The muscle and red-cell content of scavenger enzymes may correlate with fitness.

• Exercise-induced changes in oxygen-free radicals are evanescent and do not accumulate after repeated days of exercise. There is no cogent evidence that supplements of antioxidant vitamins can mitigate exercise-induced free radical formation.

IMPORTANT RESEARCH TOPICS

---

138. Tools are needed to discriminate between oxidative stress and tissue damage from exercise.
139. These tools should be employed to determine whether physical activity increases free radical formation.
140. If physical activity is shown to increase free radical formation, the roles of free radicals in the etiology of exercise-induced pathology need to be examined.

Physical Activity and the Brain

Recent evidence indicates that regional brain blood flow increases during supine dynamic exercise and that this increase is influenced by exercise intensity. The increase in regional brain blood flow during exercise is not associated with an increased glucose turnover.

Physical exercise may increase the concentrations of certain circulating endorphins. The magnitude of these changes is related to both exercise intensity and duration. The effects of increases in concentrations of these peptides is unclear, but they are known to depress pain sensitivity and to elevate pain tolerance.

IMPORTANT RESEARCH TOPICS

141. How is blood flow distributed, modified, and regulated in specific regions of the brain during different forms of exercise?
142. Is there a relationship between changes in regional blood flow and glucose turnover in specific regions of the brain?
143. Does brain substrate utilization change during exercise?
144. What endogenous substances are involved in central nervous system fatigue?
145. What are the roles of specific neuromodulators and neurotransmitters (e.g., serotonin, dopamine, norepinephrine, and gama-amino-butyric acid) in the execution and modulation of exercise?
146. Can physical activity influence incidence and/or the progression of neuropathologies such as schizophrenia, migraine, and Alzheimer's disease?

Physical Activity and Perceptual and Sensory Mechanisms

There are few data on the effects of exercise on sensation and perception. In the broader context of cognitive-motor functioning, some data show that habitually physically active individuals have more rapid motor responses than sedentary individuals.

There are few reliable data from intervention studies to show any benefit of exercise on cognitive-motor functioning in young or middle-aged subjects. In contrast, there are some data that show an improved efficiency in the perception-action cycle (i.e., response speed) in the elderly. Unfortunately, none of these studies have used methodologies which permit localization of the improved efficiency.

There are few theories underlying research in this area and most studies have been conducted in a nonsystematic fashion. Data which suggest that exercise may benefit perception-action efficiency are confounded by design problems, failure of replications, and poorly assessed dependent variables. These studies also exhibit problems in describing exercise programs, assessing fitness levels, obtaining stable cognitive-motor measures, and accounting for changes in variance estimates.

A number of studies have shown that good health is associated with efficient cognitive-motor processes. For example, some individuals who are afflicted with coronary heart disease, cerebral vascular disease and atherosclerosis exhibit impaired cognitive-motor functioning (slowed response speed). Since such diseases covary with age, much of this work has attempted to disassociate primary aging processes from the secondary declines produced by pathological conditions.

Movement speed is usually faster in physically active than in sedentary adults. Moreover, some studies on older adults who exercise regularly show better scores on psychomotor and cognitive tests (WAIS, STROOP, and Memory tests). Despite these positive results, exercise interventions have failed to improve the cognitive-motor performance of sedentary older adults consistently.

As with the evidence in young and healthy subjects, cognitive-motor research in older individuals suffers from a nonsystematic approach, with little emphasis on hypothesis-driven experiments. Further, the interpretation of the cross-sectional evidence which purports to demonstrate a benefit for older adults who are physically active can be criticized. For example, stimuli to achieve high fitness levels are highly correlated with factors which optimize cognitive-motor function (motivation, instructional set, intelligence, educational level, and socioeconomic status).

IMPORTANT RESEARCH TOPICS

147. Does physical activity affect cognitive-motor processing in young and middle-aged individuals? What are the processes and mechanisms by which exercise influences the cognitive-motor functions?
148. Does physical activity slow the rate loss of cognitive-motor processing found among the elderly? If so, what types of exercise are most effective?
149. Can physical activity restore some of the typical declines in cognitive-motor processing that are found in the elderly? If so, what types of exercise are most effective?

Physical Activity, the Nervous System, and Neural Adaptation

Our current understanding of neural adaptation to physical activity involves many aspects of human behavior. Future work should address issues related to the higher levels of neural integration within the spinal cord, as well as by supraspinal centers that initiate or modulate movement. The mammalian spinal cord can execute complex motor tasks in the absence of supraspinal control, facilitating the study of neural and muscular plasticity in spinally impaired mammals, including humans. For example, the spinal cord can regain the ability to generate stepping after the removal of supraspinal control. Further, the ability of the spinal cord to generate stepping can be modified by training in specific motor tasks.

The most useful concept underlying the neurophysiological regulation of muscle force is the "size principle," that is, the order of recruitment of motor units is inversely related to parameters associated with the size of the motor unit. This concept forms the basis of the neurophysiological phenomena that are eventually integrated to form efferent signals within each motor pool. Because virtually all movements require the recruitment of components from two or more motor pools, generalized recruitment strategies, not only within but also across motor pools, need to be identified. To understand how force output of motor units is generated, the interactive dynamics among multiple motor units and between muscle units and connective tissue-tendon-bone interfaces must be defined more clearly. For example, muscle fibers of fast motor units gradually taper in cross-sectional area and often end midfascicularly, whereas the fibers of a slow unit appear to be more uniform in size throughout their length and to extend the fascicle boundaries.

Neurophysiological, morphological, and behavioral studies suggest that neural pathways involved in the control of movement are, in part, activity (impulse) dependent. For example, there are clear changes that occur in the spinal stretch reflex in reponse to short- and long-term exposure to microgravity. Moreover, postural deficiencies remain for hours to weeks following spaceflight. Other examples of neuroplasticity include: (a) evidence that monkeys can enhance or depress the monosynaptic reflexes, (b) decerebrated cats can learn to modify their stepping to avoid an obstacle, and (c) the cat spinal cord can be trained to either perform stepping or to stand without a supraspinal input. Activity dependency is a factor in the neonatal development of sensory as well as motor systems. This activity dependency is evident throughout life, although the potential for adaptation decreases with age. Changes vary from modulations of ionic transport properties in specific receptor channels to anatomical modifications of neural pathways. Significant progress is being made toward understanding long-term potentiation, memory, learning, and the role of excitatory amino acids in producing these functional modifications.

Although it has been shown that neuromuscular activity can affect some of the mechanical and metabolic properties of motor units, there is also considerable activity-independence of those properties. For example, a normal range of motor unit (and muscle fiber) types can persist even after six months of electrical silence. Some motor neurons and some muscle fibers can change from a slow to a fast type in response to experimental reductions of activity, whereas others are quite resistant to this adaptation.

Several studies suggest that the number of muscle fibers innervated is determined by the type of motoneuron, but this may not be activity dependent. The level of activity may be important in guiding the coordination of motor axons to a specific number and type of muscle fiber. In humans, beyond the seventh decade of life there is a progressive loss in the motoneurons innervating fast muscle fibers. It appears that orphaned muscle fibers may be reinnervated by slow motoneurons.

IMPORTANT RESEARCH TOPICS

150. Are the fundamental differences found in the architecture of fast and slow muscle units general phenomena?
151. How does the arrangement of muscle fibers affect the mechanical output of motor units?
152. To what extent are the properties of the muscle fibers activity dependent or genetically determined?
153. What are the respective roles of passive and active loading in maintaining the mechanical and metabolic properties of the muscle fiber, motor unit, and muscle?
154. What are the primary spinal cord neuromodulators and neurotransmitters associated with locomotion?

155. To what extent do the kinetics and kinematics of a movement reflect the properties of the neural pathways versus musculoskeletal design?
156. What are the morphological and neurochemical mechanisms that govern the ability of a neuronal network to learn, initiate, and control a specific motor task?
157. Is the development of coordinated motor skills in children influenced by increased physical activity?
158. Is the rate and level of recovery of coordinated motor skills in the motor-impaired affected by physical activity?

Physical Activity and Cognitive Function

Many aspects of intellectual performance have been correlated to physical activity, often with the suggestion that intellectual performance responds positively to increased levels of physical activity (chronic and/or acute). Included in the list of potential benefits are academic performance as well as intellectual functioning (e.g., memory and cognitive response). Among the wide-ranging and broad generalizations proposed, only the following conclusions seem warranted.

The beneficial effects of chronic exercise on cognitive function (i.e., memory, intelligence, reaction time) are small but consistent. Cross-sectional data comparing fit and unfit individuals indicate that fit individuals display faster reaction times. However, data regarding the beneficial impact of exercise on choice reaction time are equivocal for the elderly. Perceptual-motor training which consists of low levels of physical activity has no beneficial effect upon cognitive function.

IMPORTANT RESEARCH TOPICS

159. Are the effects of exercise upon cognitive function linear?
160. Are the effects of exercise on cognitive function general in nature or specific to certain types of cognitive activity?
161. Is exercise a practicable intervention for delaying the debilitating effects of aging on cognitive performance?

162. Do the beneficial effects of exercise on cognitive function disappear upon termination of the activity?
163. Do the effects of exercise on cognitive function generalize to children?
164. How are the effects of exercise on cognitive function best explained?

Physical Activity and Lifestyle Behavior

A "healthy lifestyle" is exemplified when an individual, within the context of his/her own individual biological restrictions and particular physical and social environment, lives a life which reflects a consistent pattern of healthy behavior. Of particular interest is the relationship of exercise to behaviors such as smoking, dietary practices including alcohol consumption, and various self-protective behaviors such as seat belt use. Although the general quality of the evidence pertaining to the relationship of physical activity and other leisure behavior is weak, certain conclusions seem warranted.

Correlational studies indicate a week inverse association of both smoking status (smoking versus nonsmoking) and smoking consumption (number of cigarettes per day), with the level of leisure-time physical activity. Retrospective and prospective observational studies of selected activity groups indicate that although active groups generally smoke less than do the inactive groups at baseline, these differences do not increase at follow-up. Although the inverse relationship of exercise and smoking has been consistently reported across both male and female populations, the reported relationship is somewhat stronger in males.

Metabolic ward research indicates that an increase of physical activity, at least to a moderate level (daily energy expenditure increased to 125% of base level), results in a corresponding increase in the food energy intake of non-obese individuals. Under similar, controlled conditions, obese individuals do not adjust their energy intake. More active individuals report better nutritional practices (e.g., lower percentage of saturated fat, more balanced diet, a good breakfast). No consistent relationship is evident between exercise and alcohol consumption.

IMPORTANT RESEARCH TOPICS

---

165. Randomized prospective intervention studies should be conducted to investigate the influence of physical activity on other lifestyle behaviors. Such studies require a clear theoretical framework, valid measures, and control for potential confounders, especially socioeconomic status.

166. Future research investigating the relationship of physical activity to other lifestyle behaviors should determine the motives underlying the pertinent behaviors, using in-depth qualitative studies, as appropriate.

167. There is a need for research that examines physical activity of various types and intensity, and takes into account the social conditions of the activity as these affect tobacco and alcohol use, in particular.

168. Research should investigate whether lifestyle change programs are more effective if they focus on specific target behaviors (e.g., physical activity) than on overall lifestyle.

169. Is the efficacy of different behavior change strategies specific to population groups (e.g., age, sex, education level) or to differing motivations?

170. What role, if any, does health-related fitness play in the relationship of physical activity to other lifestyle behaviors?

Physical Activity and Psychosocial Outcomes

Definitive statements in the research literature are hampered by inconsistent operational definitions of physical activity, psychosocial outcomes, and psychological health. Psychosocial outcomes can be of a behavioral, perceptual, affective, physiological, or cognitive nature. The current literature has focused on the anxiolytic, stress-dampening, and anti-depressant effects of exercise and physical activity (which are dealt with later). A more modest segment of the literature deals with the effects of physical activity on self-perceptions of personal efficacy, self-esteem, and psychological well-being (positive affect). These conclusions are based on this latter literature.

There is a positive relationship between exercise habits and self-esteem for both adults and children. The consistency of this association is strengthened when esteem is measured at the level of specific domains rather than globally, and where exercise is valued by the individual.

There is a positive association between acute and chronic forms of exercise and psychological well-being. This relationship is stronger when measures of positive affect are employed. However, there is no evidence that the relationship between exercise and psychological well-being holds for individuals in an overtrained state.

There is a consistent positive association between exercise and self-efficacy. This relationship holds for both acute and chronic exercise, normal and clinical populations, and for adult males and females. Some evidence exists to suggest that aerobic fitness and self-efficacy are positively related, and that the effect of exercise on positive affect is mediated by self-efficacy.

IMPORTANT RESEARCH TOPICS

---

171. What are the relationships among the positive psychosocial outcomes of self-esteem, self-efficacy, and psychological well-being as a function of exercise participation?

172. Are changes in affect and esteem a function of underlying change in self-efficacy, or are other social, psychological, biological, or environmental factors implicated?

173. What role, if any, does physical fitness play in the enhancement of positive psychosocial outcomes?

174. Longitudinal studies employing randomized designs with adequate follow-up and conceptually and psychometrically-sound measures are required to extend and replicate an understanding of the effects of exercise on positive psychosocial outcomes.

Chapter 7

Physical Activity and Fitness in Disease

Physical Activity, Fitness, and Atherosclerosis

Physical activity may influence the initiation, progression, regression, and the thrombo-embolic consequences of atherosclerosis by a variety of mechanisms. Effects on HDL provide one of several possible links between exercise and atherosclerosis.

Studies of the effects of exercise on various parameters of blood coagulation, insulin resistance and glucose intolerance, and lipoprotein metabolism are described in other sections of this statement, but there are no human studies of progression or regression of atherosclerosis as modified by exercise alone.

There are studies showing a reduction in the extent of lesion formation through exercise in experimental animals kept on atherogenic diets. There are no animal studies examining the effect of exercise on atherosclerosis induced by injury. Angiographically documented regression has been observed in studies which have included exercise as part of the therapeutic regimen.

IMPORTANT RESEARCH TOPICS

Several relevant research topics can also be found in the sections dealing with fibrinolysis, platelet aggregability, lipid metabolism, and Type II diabetes.

175. Randomized, clinical trials should be implemented to evaluate exercise alone or exercise compared to other interventions in the treatment of established atherosclerotic lesions.

176. Exercise-induced modification of atherosclerosis caused by endothelial injury should be examined in experimental animals who are not receiving dietary lipid supplements.

Physical Activity, Fitness, and Coronary Heart Disease

Sedentary living is associated with a high incidence of coronary heart disease. This observation is supported by numerous prospective studies from Europe and North America based on groups of apparently healthy individuals who were followed for fatal and nonfatal coronary heart disease for up to 20 years. The majority of studies show an inverse relationship of coronary heart disease rates across physical activity levels. There is near unanimity that physical activity provides some protection against coronary heart disease in studies that have used good or excellent epidemiological methods, including valid and reliable assessment of physical activity and comprehensive surveillance of disease endpoints. There is an approximate doubling in risk of coronary heart disease when the least active individuals are compared with their most active peers. The association of inactivity to coronary heart disease is not due solely to the confounding influences of other favorable lifestyle behaviors.

Several recent studies have assessed physical fitness at baseline by either maximal or sub-maximal exercise testing. There is an inverse gradient of coronary heart disease death rates across fitness groups. The gradient across the distribution of exposure seems much steeper for the fitness-coronary heart disease studies than for activity-coronary heart disease studies. The relative risk for coronary heart disease in the least active compared to most active is approximately 2.0. When fitness is the exposure variable, relative risks as high as 8.0 are seen when comparing least fit with most fit individuals. Although the reasons for these differences in relative risk between activity and fitness studies are unclear, there may be less misclassification in the fitness studies, because habitual physical activity is difficult to assess reliably. Physical fitness is an excellent overall marker of physical activity and may provide precision for studies on the physical activity-coronary heart disease hypothesis.

Data on the relationship between activity and coronary heart disease in women are less convincing than the data from studies on men. However, the relationship between fitness and cardiovascular disease mortality show similar relative risks in men and women when individuals with low and high fitness levels are compared. Possibly, physical activity has not been assessed accurately in women because most activity assessment techniques have been developed for use with men.

There is a strong inverse gradient of coronary heart disease rates across activity or fitness levels. Low levels of activity or fitness precede the development of coronary heart disease in healthy individuals. Results are consistent within and across populations, and the epidemiological findings are plausible and coherent with the results from clinical and experimental investigations. The current literature thus strongly supports the concept that sedentary living habits increase the risk for coronary heart disease.

IMPORTANT RESEARCH TOPICS

177. What are the specific type, intensity, duration, frequency, and total amount of physical activity required to prevent coronary heart disease?
178. What is the role of physical activity in the prevention of coronary heart disease in women and minority groups?
179. What is the relative importance of lifetime and current patterns of physical activity with respect to the risk of coronary heart disease?
180. Is the risk of coronary heart disease reduced in sedentary, middle-aged, and older men and women if they convert to a more active way of life?
181. What are the independent and interactive contributions of physical activity and fitness to the risk of coronary heart disease?

Physical Activity, Fitness, and CHD Rehabilitation

Cardiac rehabilitation is defined by the World Health Organization as "the sum of activities required to ensure cardiac patients the best possible physical, mental, and social conditions so that they may, by their own efforts, resume as normal a place as possible in the life of the community . . . and that . . . rehabilitation cannot be regarded as an isolated form of therapy, but must be integrated into the whole treatment of which it constitutes only one facet."

As a general principle, low-level physical activity should begin within the first few days of infarction. Periodic exposure to gravitational stress during the early stages of convalescence decreases the complications of bed rest. Prescribed exercise should be gradually increased throughout the period of hospitalization, until it approximates the level of physical activity required for resumption of self-care at home. Such a plan prepares the patient for a predischarge exercise test, which can be used in addition to clinical features to stratify the risk of a recurrence. Early mobilization has no adverse effects on short- or long-term morbidity and mortality.

Among patients requiring supervised exercise, less than 30% require continuous electrocardiogram monitoring. In short-term (8 to 12 week) studies of supervised exercise programs, exercise capacity improved whether the patients were in a usual care or active intervention group. However, the exercise groups typically had a 20 to 25% greater exercise capacity than the usual care treatment groups. Low-risk survivors may not need a closely supervised cardiac rehabilitation program and may graduate directly to rehabilitation at home.

Limited data suggest that patients with anterior Q-wave myocardial infarctions might develop detrimental ventricular shape distortion after exercise training, but this has not been verified. In general, patients with ventricular dysfunction improve exercise capacity from exercise training. Older post-myocardial infarction patients seem to benefit from exercise training as much as younger ones.

Several meta-analyses of randomized trials of cardiac rehabilitation involving thousands of patients have demonstrated a 20% reduction of risk for total mortality, and a 25% reduction in the risk for fatal reinfarction. However, most of these studies have involved structured exercise programs continued for long periods post myocardial infarction. Current estimates are that the incidence of cardiac arrest is approximately one death per 100,000 patient-hours of exercise in supervised cardiac rehabilitation programs. Cardiac rehabilitation improves functional capacity and reduces symptoms in patients after surgery for coronary artery bypass and cardiac transplantation.

182. Does exercise training improve the quality of life and survival in patients with heart failure?
183. Can exercise training in patients with coronary heart disease improve myocardial perfusion and function?
184. Does cardiac rehabilitation lower health care costs and improve psychosocial outcomes?

Physical Activity, Fitness, and Stroke

Stroke incidence and mortality are major public health problems in developed countries. Atherosclerosis is thought to be the underlying pathologic cause of most thromboembolic (ischemic) strokes, whereas hypertensive disease is the major pathologic determinant of hemorrhagic stroke. There is little direct evidence relating physical activity and/ or physical fitness to the risk of thromboembolic or hemorrhagic stroke. Data from animal models are scarce.

Data relating physical activity to the risk of stroke are equivocal. Weaknesses of study design, including incomplete or non-existent control for potential confounding variables, often temporally incorrect and inadequate measures of physical activity, and potentially incomplete case definition and ascertainment, contribute to equivocal conclusions. No published studies have examined physical fitness and the risk of stroke.

Physical activity and fitness could be related to a lower risk of thromboembolic stroke either directly or indirectly (by influencing other factors thought to increase the risk of stroke). The potential mechanisms for any direct influence on atherosclerotic plaque or lesions in the arteries to the brain are unknown.

Physical activity or fitness may also alter the risk of hemorrhagic stroke. Such alteration may be based on blood pressure effects and the intensity of physical activity. Moderate exercise lowers resting blood pressure and may thus lower the risk of hemorrhagic stroke. High-intensity exercise could conceivably induce hemorrhagic stroke and such a tendency has been found in stroke-prone hypertensive rats.

185. Is there an association between habitual physical activity and/or fitness and the risk of stroke?
186. Is there an increased risk of stroke during acute, intense physical activity, and if so, is this risk influenced by the type of exercise?
187. What is the role that physical activity plays in atherosclerotic plaque formation and regression?
188. What is the role that physical activity plays in atherosclerotic plaque rupture?
189. What is the interaction of physical activity and/or fitness with other established risk factors for stroke?

Physical Activity, Fitness, and Peripheral Vascular Disease

More than 30 studies, almost all without any control group, have documented that regular exercise increases physical performance capacity in patients with peripheral vascular disease of the lower extremities. Both the walking distance before the onset of claudication and the maximum walking distance are increased. Gains in performance have ranged from less than 50% to more than 1,000%. The increase in performance is unrelated to the extent of disease or the duration of training. The extent of ischemic stimulus imposed during the training may be a critical factor.

The mechanism responsible for the improvement in performance is unknown. There is evidence to support the development of collateral vessels, an increase in maximum blood flow, a redistribution of flow within the ischemic leg and an increase in blood fluidity. Biochemical changes including an increase in aerobic enzymes have been reported, but these changes are unlikely to be major factors in the increase of performance because of the deficient oxygen supply.

190. Does regular physical activity prevent the development or delay the presentation of peripheral vascular disease?

191. What are the stimuli and mechanisms responsible for adaptation to exercise training in patients with peripheral vascular disease?
192. What is the most effective exercise prescription for patients with peripheral vascular disease?
193. Does regular exercise have an effect on atherosclerosis and on related risk factors in patients with peripheral vascular disease?
194. How do the short- and long-term results of regular exercise compare with other hygienic, medical, and invasive interventions in patients with peripheral vascular disease?
195. What is the best exercise testing protocol for evaluating the severity of peripheral vascular disease?

Physical Activity, Fitness, and Blood Pressure

Hypertension is a risk factor for heart disease and stroke, and a major public health problem. At the present time, the primary risk factors for high blood pressure have been identified as genetic predisposition, advanced age, high body mass index, excessive sodium intake, increased consumption of alcohol, and lack of regular exercise. Blood pressure measurements during exercise have not proven to be good independent predictors of either future hypertension in normotensive populations or of the incidence of cardiovascular events in hypertensives.

Studies in humans and animals have repeatedly demonstrated that normotensive and hypertensive populations exhibit a postexercise decrease in resting blood pressure below preexercise levels. This may persist for several hours. The mechanism and the significance of such observations are not known.

Most cross-sectional epidemiological studies show an inverse relationship between resting blood pressure and fitness levels, habitual physical activity, or exercise. However, in the majority of studies, the difference between the most and least physically active or fit subjects was seldom more than 5 mmHg. In longitudinal studies, physical activity and fitness were inversely related to the development of hypertension.

When the effects of chronic endurance exercise were examined with experimental designs that included nonexercising subjects or control conditions, 48 groups of "healthy" normotensive and hypertensive subjects were identified, mostly men. These studies indicate that relative to controls, endurance training was associated with a mean reduction of systolic/diastolic blood pressure of 3/3 mmHg in the groups with a normal average pressure; of 6/7 mmHg in borderline hypertensives; and of 10/8 mmHg in hypertensives. In the genetic spontaneously hypertensive rat, endurance training studies have consistently demonstrated that trained rats will have resting systolic or mean arterial pressures that are 10 mmHg lower than their untrained controls. In adult hypertensive rats, the lower resting pressures of trained populations are because training prevents the increase in pressure that occurs with aging.

Endurance training in humans has not consistently reduced the blood pressure response during dynamic exercise. Monitoring of blood pressure during 24 hours showed that a training-induced decrease of blood pressure during the daytime was not observed during the night when the subjects were sleeping.

The hemodynamic mechanism underlying the hypotensive effect of endurance training remains controversial as the observed decrease in blood pressure could be due to a reduction of cardiac output and/or systemic vascular resistance. Reductions in circulating norepinephrine concentrations are associated with decreases in pressure.

Most studies indicate that strength-training does not lead to persistent changes in blood pressure; some have found limited decreases. However, any hypotensive effect seems smaller than the effect that can be achieved by dynamic aerobic training.

IMPORTANT RESEARCH TOPICS

196. What mechanisms are responsible for the acute reduction in resting blood pressure after exercise?
197. What is the optimal exercise prescription for the hypertensive patient?
198. What mechanisms are responsible for the reductions in resting and exercise blood pressures observed in endurance-trained hypertensive patients?
199. How does endurance training compare and interact with other nonpharmacological interventions and with pharmacological treatments of hypertensive patients?

200. What are the risks and benefits of weight-resistive exercises for hypertensive patients?
201. What is the role of physical activity in the prevention of hypertension and its sequelae?

Physical Activity, Fitness, and Type I Diabetes

There are few well-conducted, randomized controlled studies of habitual activity in Type I diabetes, but those available suggest that physical activity has both psychological and physiological benefits and that these apply to both diabetic and nondiabetic subjects. Exercise training increases insulin sensitivity, and may reduce insulin requirements in insulin-treated diabetics. Exercise may also have beneficial effects on the cardiovascular system and on lipoprotein profiles. However, no conclusive evidence exists that glycemic control is improved. Therefore, exercise is not recommended for the improvement of glycemia; rather, it should be recommended in the uncomplicated, well-controlled Type I diabetic, for the same reasons as for a nondiabetic individual.

Type I diabetics should not be discouraged from engaging in sport or recreational activities on the basis of their insulin dependency. However, patients should be instructed in self-monitoring, because their glycemic response to exercise is often abnormal, depending on the degree of insulinization achieved with their current insulin regimen.

In nondiabetic subjects, plasma glucose levels do not change during mild to moderate exercise; the exercise-induced increase in glucose uptake is matched by a corresponding increase in glucose production. In contrast to nondiabetic individuals, the subcutaneous absorption of insulin does not decrease and may even increase during physical activity in insulin-treated diabetics, particularly if the injected limb is physically active. Therefore, the increase in glucose uptake induced by physical activity may not be matched by a corresponding increase in glucose production, with a resulting acute hypoglycemia. Hypoglycemia can also occur in insulin-treated diabetic subjects several hours after physical activity, because of the exercise-induced increase in insulin sensitivity.

Underinsulinization also results in abnormalities of fuel homeostasis during physical activity. If the insulin deficiency is substantial, the exercise-induced increase in glucose uptake is attenuated and the increase in glucose production results in a worsening of hyperglycemia.

Intensive physical activity can be more deleterious to diabetic control than moderate activity of similar duration. The normal hyperglycemic response to exhausting exercise is exaggerated even in well-controlled Type I diabetics, who are unable to respond to hyperglycemia with increased insulin secretion.

With proper instructions and careful monitoring, most uncomplicated Type I diabetics can exercise safely. Blood glucose self-monitoring is mandatory before any unplanned, prolonged or vigorous physical activity. Exercising Type I diabetics should always have glucose reading strips, and a readily absorbed form of carbohydrate available. It is very important that they monitor their blood glucose concentrations prior to, during, and after exercise and adjust their carbohydrate intake accordingly. Metabolic control is more easily achieved and the risk of hypoglycemia is lessened if exercise is carefully planned.

Diabetics treated with conventional therapy (one or two daily injections with or without short-acting insulin) should not engage in physical activity at the peak of action of the injected insulin. Exercise is best carried out postprandially in these patients. The overall risk of hypoglycemia is greater with intensified insulin treatment (multiple injection regimens or Continuous Subcutaneous Insulin Infusion) than with conventional treatment. However, the risk of exercise-related hypoglycemic events can be lessened by reduction of premeal insulin boluses and basal insulin infusion. Patients treated with Continuous Subcutaneous Insulin Infusion or with a regimen of daily insulin boluses and bed-time intermediate insulin can safely exercise in both the postabsorptive and the postprandial state.

Clinical impressions and common sense suggest that caution should be used in recommending exercise to diabetic patients with the following:

• Proliferative retinopathy, because of the possibility of intraocular hemorrhages and retinal detachment during heavy exercise.

• Severe peripheral neuropathy or vascular disease (exercise can then traumatize the insensitive or ischemic foot).

• Autonomic neuropathy with postural hypotension (since heavy exercise might precipitate hypotensive episodes or cardiac arrhythmia). With less severe autonomic neuropathy, particular attention should be paid to the maintenance of proper hydration.

• Diabetic nephropathy with heavy proteinuria (for the possibility that exercise-induced dehydration and increase in proteinuria may precipitate acute renal failure).

• Coronary heart disease in the immediate post-infarct period (for the possibility that the elevated incidence of arrhythmia in diabetes may be further increased by exercise) and in patients with unstable angina or moderate to severe heart failure. In patients with stable coronary heart disease and in the later phases of postinfarct rehabilitation, exercise is recommended, but careful preexercise evaluation, and judicious and supervised training programs are indicated.

• Cerebrovascular disease with recurrent transient ischemic attacks (for the possibility that perfusion of the brain may be jeopardized by an exercise-induced lowering of systemic vascular resistance).

IMPORTANT RESEARCH TOPICS

202. What are the independent roles of insulin, glycemia, and the free fatty acid-glucose cycle in the exercise-induced rise in glucose uptake, clearance, oxidation, and storage? And, what is the status of glucose transporters?

203. What are the mechanisms of alteration in counter-regulatory responses observed during physical activity in Type I diabetics with and without autonomic neuropathy?

204. How do the metabolic effects of moderate and strenuous physical activity differ in Type I diabetes?

205. What is the antiatherogenic potential of the reduction in insulin dosage induced by exercise training in diabetic patients?

206. Long-term controlled studies in large populations are needed to evaluate the risks and benefits of acute and chronic exercise in diabetics.

207. There needs to be objective assessment of the risks of exercise in patients with diabetic complications, in particular, for those with proliferative retinopathy.

Physical Activity, Fitness, and Type II Diabetes

Type II diabetes or non-insulin-dependent diabetes mellitus comprises some 80% of diabetic patients. Its prevalence in most western countries is 2 to 3% and, in some epidemiological studies, one case is undiagnosed for every case that is known. In some populations like the Pima Indians in Arizona, the prevalence of Type II diabetes is over 30%. Non-insulin-dependent diabetes mellitus comprises a heterogeneous group of conditions, is more prevalent among obese persons, and is associated with an impairment of insulin secretion plus resistance to insulin. These two abnormalities seem linked in a vicious circle; chronic hyperglycemia impairs both insulin secretion and insulin sensitivity ("glucose toxicity"). The major site of insulin resistance appears to be in the skeletal muscle, particularly in the mechanisms leading to muscle glycogen accumulation. There is a strong hereditary component in Type II diabetes, but in contrast to Type I diabetes, there is no evidence that Type II diabetes mellitus is linked with the genes of the major histocompatibility region (such as Class II antigens of the HLA system).

Several studies in healthy volunteers have shown that physical activity and exercise training increase insulin sensitivity. Furthermore, in middle-aged individuals, regular exercise tends to improve tolerance to orally ingested glucose and to modify favorably several recognized risk factors for cardiovascular disease such as excess total and abdominal fat, adverse plasma lipoprotein levels, and mild-to-moderate arterial hypertension.

Numerous descriptive studies have shown that the prevalence of Type II diabetes mellitus is higher in inactive urban than in active rural populations. Furthermore, cross-sectional studies have shown that the prevalence of Type II diabetes (or abnormal glucose tolerance) is greater among sedentary individuals than among their active counterparts, independent of age and body mass index. Two epidemiological studies of large populations have shown that in both men and women the relative risk of developing Type II diabetes is lower in subjects who exercise regularly. This protective benefit of exercise is especially pronounced in persons with a high body mass index, a history of arterial hypertension, or a family history of diabetes. Thus, the concept has emerged that increased physical activity is associated with a reduced incidence of Type II diabetes. The prevalence of insulin resistance in non-diabetic sedentary individuals (~25% of adults) is such that an improvement in insulin sensitivity, produced by regular aerobic exercise training, may reduce the risk of non-insulin-dependent diabetes in a significant portion of the population.

Many studies have included physical activity as part of the treatment of Type II diabetes mellitus. Potential beneficial effects of physical training include lower blood glucose and glycosylated hemoglobin levels, lower fasting and postprandial plasma insulin levels, increased insulin sensitivity, favorable changes in plasma lipid profiles, increased cardiovascular fitness and physical work capacity, increased antithrombotic activity, and an improved self-esteem and sense of well being. However, exercise in Type II diabetic patients is not without risk or contraindications similar to those discussed for Type I diabetes. Practical considerations include: preexercise evaluation, the nature of the exercise prescription itself and appropriate precautions.

The literature indicates that exercise has a definite potential to improve glucose tolerance and reduce the insulin response in patients with impaired glucose tolerance or very early non-insulin-dependent diabetes mellitus. Evidence for exercise-induced improvement in metabolic control in more severe forms of non-insulin-dependent diabetes mellitus is scant. However, the exercise programs evaluated to date have generally involved low to moderate intensities of exercise, prescribed for only a few weeks. The amount of exercise required for improvements in blood glucose control is unknown and may be greater than the minimal amount needed to improve cardiovascular fitness. The feasibility of using exercise training in this population may also be lower than for the general population. Even when an exercise program is feasible in a given patient, compliance is not always achieved.

IMPORTANT RESEARCH TOPICS

208. Is there an optimal combination of exercise mode, intensity, duration, and frequency for preventing Type II diabetes or improving control in patients with manifest Type II diabetes?
209. To what extent are the effects of exercise independent of changes in body mass?
210. How does exercise improve insulin sensitivity in Type II diabetes?
211. What are the risks of an exercise program in Type II diabetes?
212. To what extent does the risk/benefit ratio of physical training programs differ between various subgroups of diabetic patients?
213. How long do the beneficial metabolic and/or cardiovascular effects of an exercise program persist after the cessation of physical activity, and how is this persistence modified by the state of training of the individual?
214. How can one improve the compliance of Type II diabetic patients to exercise programs?

Physical Activity, Fitness, and Moderate Obesity

Obesity, a condition characterized by an excessive percentage of body fat, results from an energy intake that exceeds the habitual energy expenditure. Physical activity is an important variable to consider in understanding and treating obesity since it is the principal discretionary component of energy expenditure and it can modify both energy intake and body composition.

It is likely that physical inactivity contributes to the development of obesity in some individuals and that activity helps prevent obesity in others. Studies in rodents have demonstrated that both inactivity and exercise cessation lead to an increased body fat content. Moreover, exercise can attenuate the increase in body fat that would otherwise occur when rodents are given high-fat diets.

The cause and effect relationship between inactivity and obesity is less clearly established for humans. Most data suggest that many obese persons engage in low levels of habitual physical activity relative to their non-obese counterparts. However, it is not possible to conclude that physical inactivity has caused the obesity. Prospective research using better techniques to quantify physical activity is needed to demonstrate a causal relationship between inactivity and obesity.

It may be erroneous to target physical inactivity as the sole cause of obesity. For example, even if an individual displays a reduced level of physical activity, obesity could only result if the energy intake was inappropriately high for the individual's overall level of energy expenditure. Thus, obesity would result not from inactivity alone but from a failure to match energy intake with energy expenditure.

When an obese person begins an exercise program, a condition of negative energy balance develops unless there is compensation (increased intake, decreased spontaneous activity) for the energy expended in exercise. Most data suggest moderately obese humans do not show complete energy compensation when they exercise. The negative energy balance thus produces a loss of body mass and/or a change in body composition, the extent of which is determined by the magnitude of the negative energy balance.

Exercise and exercise training may increase total daily energy expenditure in multiple ways. Initially, the increase is due largely to the increase of energy expenditure during the exercise bout. Any increase in postexercise energy expenditure is not likely to be significant with the moderate intensities of exercise usually used to treat obesity. With sustained and repeated bouts of exercise, there may be an increase in fat-free mass, which in turn, would increase resting energy expenditure. Neither an acute bout of exercise nor the level of aerobic fitness appears to alter the resting energy expenditure (after accounting for fat-free mass).

Exercise increases lipid oxidation and generally produces some reduction in body fat stores. The loss of body fat is greater the more exercise is undertaken and (for a given dose of exercise) the higher the body fat content of the person beginning exercise. Changes in body composition are somewhat dependent on the mode of exercise, but decreases in body fat occur with both aerobic exercise and resistance training.

Exercise alone is often dismissed as ineffective in treating obesity. A major reason is the small energy deficit produced by exercise in relation to the large energy deficit that can be induced by food restriction programs. The effectiveness of exercise as a treatment for obesity has not been adequately evaluated in studies using sustained exercise for long periods of time. It is difficult to maintain exercise compliance in obese subjects over very long periods of time. The weight loss produced by exercise alone does not produce the decline of resting energy expenditure seen with food restriction.

There is no reason to conclude from existing data that exercise is not at least additive to food restriction in terms of producing fat loss. Some of the confusion in the literature is due to inappropriate outcome expectations. Few studies have evaluated the extent of fat loss due to exercise in relation to the estimated energy deficit produced by exercise.

Regular exercise can alter fuel oxidation, and exercise has been suggested to modify the composition of the weight loss produced by food restriction alone. Much data suggest that exercise may increase fat loss and decrease the loss of fat-free mass. Many studies show a greater total fat loss with exercise and food restriction than with food restriction alone, despite similar changes of body weight. This benefit of exercise remains controversial, and may depend on the mode of exercise used and the duration of the exercise program.

Food restriction induces a decline in energy expenditure along with a decline in body mass. There is currently no indication that exercise prevents this decline. However, if exercise preserves fat-free mass, this could result in a higher resting energy expenditure following weight loss than would occur with food restriction alone.

Persons who are successful in achieving and maintaining a reduction in body weight are highly likely to be exercisers. It is not clear, however, if or how exercise provides an advantage in weight maintenance. It is possible that persons who exercise are also those who are most successful in making permanent lifestyle changes (e.g., modifying diet).

The risks of using exercise with a moderately obese population are small and consist primarily of musculoskeletal injuries due to beginning exercise at excessive intensities. Although the benefits of exercise in the treatment of obesity remain somewhat controversial, the potential benefits far outweigh the risks. It would seem prudent to include exercise in an obesity treatment program. Exercise increases the overall size of the energy deficit, increases lipid oxidation, and may increase relative fat loss. It also remains a good predictor of long-term success in weight reduction.

IMPORTANT RESEARCH TOPICS

215. Does physical inactivity cause obesity in human beings?
216. What are the mechanisms involved in matching energy intake and energy expenditure, and how are these affected by exercise and by exercise training?
217. How much energy compensation occurs when moderately obese humans begin an exercise program? Does this change over time?
218. What modes of exercise are most effective in reducing body fat content and increasing fat-free mass?
219. What are the mechanisms whereby exercise provides an advantage in the long-term maintenance of a reduced body weight?

220. Under what conditions does the combination of exercise and food restriction alter the composition of any weight that is lost?

Physical Activity, Fitness, and Severe Obesity

Severe obesity should be considered separately from moderate obesity, as adipocyte hyperplasia accompanies severe obesity. Adipocyte hyperplasia is associated with resistance to weight loss by lifestyle modification (diet, exercise, and behavioral modification). The 1991 National Institutes of Health Consensus Development Conference on Surgery for Severe Obesity defined severe obesity as a body mass index (BMI) of 40 or above, or a BMI of 35 or above if associated with complications. There are an extremely limited number of studies evaluating exercise in severe obesity as defined by these BMI values.

Conclusions from studies evaluating effects of exercise training on body mass and body composition in the severely obese are conflicting. Exercise training preferentially reduces body fat, while preserving fat-free mass. The degree of obesity and the type, intensity, frequency, and duration of exercise all affect weight loss. The limited ability of some severely obese individuals to exercise sufficiently may limit the effects of increased physical activity upon body mass, composition, or metabolic variables. Given the slow rate of weight loss with exercise and some degree of energy compensation by the subjects, the length of the studies was generally insufficient to expect major differences in body mass.

Most studies that have evaluated insulin levels and/or insulin sensitivity with exercise in the severely obese have shown improvements, although some have found no effect. Any effects on glucose tolerance are minimal, and several studies show no effect. Resting norepinephrine levels are often increased in severely obese individuals, and in general, such levels are decreased by weight loss because of exercise training or dieting. Lipoprotein profiles may improve with exercise training, even in the absence of weight loss.

Severely obese people have poor levels of health-related fitness. Strenuous exercise may be more uncomfortable for the very obese than for the general population, and this could contribute to the poor adherence to exercise programs reported in such populations. The occurrence of arthritis, venous statis lesions, thermal stress, and skin rashes in the severely obese also limit their exercise tolerance. Most available studies have shown modest increases in exercise endurance and maximum aerobic power in severely obese subjects after participation in an exercise training program.

IMPORTANT RESEARCH TOPICS

Additional studies comparing exercise training in the severely obese versus control, or moderately obese subjects should address the following questions.

221. Do the severely obese form a separate subgroup in terms of their response to an exercise training program?
222. Are there sex differences in the metabolic profiles and in the response to treatment of severely obese individuals?
223. How can compliance of the severely obese to an exercise regimen be improved?
224. What is the relative importance of the various components of the exercise prescription for the severely obese, including: type, intensity, duration, and frequency of effort?
225. Can exercise be used for long-term maintenance of weight loss in the severely obese? Is there a role for a combination of exercise and drugs in the induction or maintenance of weight loss?
226. How do dietary energy and macronutrient content affect the ability of severely obese subjects to exercise, the outcome of weight-loss programs, and the complications of their obesity?
227. Does pre- or postsurgery exercise alter the outcome of obesity surgery in any way?

Physical Activity, Fitness, and Osteoarthritis

Osteoarthritis is the most common of over 100 types of arthritis, but it has a poorly understood multifactorial etiology. It leads to cartilaginous degeneration and is associated with clinical symptoms. Factors important in pathogenesis include genetic predisposition, trauma, inflammation, and biochemical characteristics. Immunologic events, occupational and environmental influences, and recreational patterns also have possible importance. The physical characteristics of the participant, biomechanical factors, age, sex, hormonal influences, state of nutrition, characteristics of the playing surface, unique features of particular sports, and the duration and intensity of effort can all influence the effects of exercise participation. A uniform view of the clinical, radiologic, and pathologic criteria that can be used to define osteoarthritis has not yet been reached. This has limited understanding of osteoarthritis and has created difficulties in analyzing the effects of exercise and sport-related activities on the risk of developing osteoarthritis.

There is currently little definitive information about the impact of physical activity on the development of osteoarthritis. Data on the relationship between exercise and osteoarthritis from animal studies have been inconsistent. In humans, numerous retrospective studies have alleged a possible relationship between sports participation and osteoarthritis. They include observations of osteoarthritis developing in joints subjected to sport-related stresses in wrestlers, boxers, baseball pitchers, cyclists, sports parachutists, cricketers, gymnasts, ballet dancers, soccer players, and American football players. Similarly, evidence that osteoarthritis follows repetitive occupational activities is inconsistent and inconclusive. Most of these data are difficult to evaluate because of methodological inadequacies.

Observations generally suggest that individuals who have run long distances for many years without clinical discomfort have not developed osteoarthritis at a rate that differs from nonrunner populations. Those individuals with underlying anatomic and/or biomechanical abnormalities appear to be at greater risk of subsequent development of osteoarthritis, and such observations seem valid for other sports activities as well. Limited data suggest that physical activity (carried out within the limits of comfort, putting joints through the normal range of motion, and without underlying joint abnormality) does not lead to joint injury, even if pursued over many years. Preliminary studies of therapeutic exercise programs for selected patients with rheumatoid arthritis and osteoarthritis have suggested clinical benefits.

IMPORTANT RESEARCH TOPICS

228. Further studies should define and quantify the physical stress imposed by various activities carefully. Future investigations of exercise and osteoarthritis require appropriate study and control populations. Observations should be of sufficient duration and sample size sufficient to provide definitive information. Studies are needed using standardized clinical and radiologic assessments of joint degeneration, with objective quantification of the patients' functional status, and an assessment of other risk factors. These are difficult studies to conduct, and unfortunately may never be done.

Physical Activity, Fitness, and Osteoporosis

Weight-bearing or resisted physical activity is essential for bone health. Without gravitational or mechanical loading on the axial and appendicular skeleton, there is a rapid and marked loss of bone density. Whether the generalized decrease in physical activity as one ages has a cumulative negative impact on bone mass is unknown. However, there is ample evidence that active individuals have a greater skeletal mass than those who are inactive. There are also data to support the concept that those who are sedentary can increase bone mass by becoming more physically active.

Exercise may be most effective in maximizing bone mass in young adults and maintaining bone mass during the mature adult years. On average, active people of all ages have a higher bone-mineral density than those who are sedentary. Data from cross-sectional studies indicate that active women and men less than 50 years of age average, respectively, 8% and 10% higher vertebral bone mineral density than their inactive peers. On the other hand, longitudinal data for the effect of exercise on lumbar bone mineral density in this age group are less numerous, and certainly less impressive, with changes ranging from −12 to 8%. This discrepancy may be due to the choice of physical activity and details of the exercise protocol rather than to the potential osteogenic effect that exercise might have on bone.

The positive effect of exercise on bone is also observed in postmenopausal women and older men. Cross-sectional studies show that active women have a higher bone mass than sedentary women (+7%). When sedentary older women participate in long-term physical activity programs (> 8 months) there is usually a slight increase in their lumbar bone mineral density, ranging from 1 to 8%, depending on the type of activity that is undertaken. However, the absolute level attained remains well below that of young normal women.

The most important question is whether the exercise-induced changes can decrease the risk of osteoporotic fractures by increasing bone density, by modifying bone microarchitectural, or by decreasing the likelihood of falls. Three epidemiologic studies report fewer hip fractures among men and women with a history of physical activity than in less active groups, but the studies were limited in their control of confounding factors. A conclusive assessment of the protective effect of exercise thus remains to be done.

Five general principles should be considered in planning or evaluating an exercise program to promote bone health:

- The Principle of Specificity: exercise provides a local osteogenic effect.
- The Principle of Overload: there must be a progressive increase in the intensity of the exercise for continued improvement.
- The Principle of Reversibility: the positive effect of exercise on bone would be lost if the exercise program were to be discontinued.
- The Principle of Initial Values: those who have the lowest bone mass have the greatest potential for improvement.
- The Principle of Diminishing Returns: as the biological ceiling of bone density is approached, more and more effort is required to obtain further gain.

In spite of its beneficial effect on bone, there is no evidence that exercise can substitute for hormone replacement therapy as a means of preventing bone loss in the early postmenopausal period. Experience with young hypoestrogenic athletes (usually with a negative energy balance) demonstrates that the positive effect of exercise on bone is greatly diminished if estrogen levels are subnormal despite rigorous activity. Physical activity can be an important adjunct to any hormone replacement therapy that is required and may help older individuals to improve coordination, balance, and muscle strength. These effects may decrease the likelihood of fracture independent of bone mass by preventing falls and/or minimizing the trauma of a fall.

IMPORTANT RESEARCH TOPICS

229. How do the general principles of training apply to the skeletal system? What is the magnitude, the frequency, and the distribution of an effective load; how are different parts of the skeleton affected; and what is the time course of the response?

230. How does exercise interact with endogenous hormones, and what biochemical markers reflect the effect of this interaction upon bone?

231. What is the appropriate exercise prescription for maintaining and increasing bone mass during childhood, adolescence, maturity, and the early and late postmenopausal years?

232. What are the interactive effects on bone mass of increased physical activity, nutrition, and pharmacologic interventions?

233. How does vertebral collapse affect other physiologic systems such as cardiovascular and respiratory function, and what is the potential of physical activity to prevent or ameliorate such adverse effects?

234. How might exercise affect structural factors other than bone mass which might decrease the risk of osteoporotic fractures?

Physical Activity, Fitness, and Back Pain

Back pain is a syndrome typically identified by individual self-report. Because of the subjective nature of back pain, interpretation of existing data is problematic. Methods for evaluation of "back fitness" are much less standardized than for cardiorespiratory function. The reproducibility is best for isometric trunk muscle tests.

A history of heavy physical work, forward bending, static work, torsion, and in particular, heavy lifting are strongly correlated with the incidence of low back pain. The causal role of sedentary occupations is less clear and often has not been addressed properly in epidemiological studies.

There is a lack of adequate data regarding the relationship between physical activity or sport participation and back pain in the general population. Various reports suggest that young athletes with low back pain have underlying structural problems. Anecdotal data suggest that back pain in sport is also caused by acute traumatic injury or effects of cumulative overuse.

Cadaver studies indicate that physical activity strengthens both the vertebrae and the intervertebral discs. Symmetric disc degeneration is associated with sedentary work, and vertebral osteophytosis is related to heavy work. Movement facilitates the nutrition of the intervertebral disc. However, other factors, like smoking, also influence disc degeneration.

A reduction of the amount of weight lifted and other ergonomic modifications of the work site can reduce the risk of certain types of occupational low back pain. The possible contributions of trunk muscular strength and endurance, trunk flexibility, and cardiovascular fitness are still questionable.

There is no unanimity as to the most appropriate treatment for existing low back pain. Trunk exercise rehabilitation programs seem beneficial in the treatment of both acute and chronic low back pain. The benefit apparently depends on the dosage rather than the use of dynamic versus isometric or extension versus flexion exercises. No randomized studies have demonstrated the superiority of the multidisciplinary treatment in comparison to exercise alone.

IMPORTANT RESEARCH TOPICS

235. A systematic approach is needed to address factors which potentially contribute to low back pain.
236. Randomized intervention studies are needed in which one or more aspects of lifting techniques are modified in one group of individuals to test the value of such changes in work site practice.
237. Interaction between physical fitness programs and other important factors, like psychosocial issues such as job responsibility and job satisfaction, should be investigated to avoid an overly-narrow focus on single-factor etiology.

238. The role of physical activity, muscular performance, and cardiovascular fitness in the prediction and prevention of back pain needs further elucidation.
239. Further research is needed in order to answer the question of intensity versus type of exercise in the treatment and prevention of back pain.
240. Standardization of dynamic trunk muscle function tests is required.

Physical Activity, Fitness, and Chronic Lung Disease

Patients with obstructive and restrictive lung disease have impaired pulmonary-mechanical function and inefficiencies of pulmonary gas exchange. This imposes increased ventilatory demands upon a system with limited response capabilities. Consequently, the tolerable range of work rates is constrained.

In obstructive pulmonary diseases, the increased flow-resistive work of breathing increases the oxygen consumption, CO_2 output and blood flow demands of the respiratory muscles, increasing the propensity to shortness of breath. Shortness of breath can be further exacerbated by hypoxemia. An increased dispersion of ventilation to perfusion ratios results in increased dead space to tidal volume ratio and arterial hypoxemia. The latter, in addition to provoking dyspnea, often results in hyperventilation with a decreased arterial CO_2 pressure. The consequence is an increased ventilatory demand for a given work rate.

The maximum attainable ventilation and the maximum achievable airflow are both reduced in obstructive lung disease. When the exercise ventilation approaches the maximal attainable ventilation, the exercise airflow encroaches upon (and may exceed) the outer limits of the patient's maximum expiratory flow-volume curve. This mechanical limitation is typically accompanied by a high rating of dyspnea, constraining further increases in work rate. Consequently, the peak O_2 intake, heart rate and blood lactate are all typically low during maximum exercise. When expiratory airflow is the dominant cause of functional impairment, the duration of inspiration can be shortened to prolong the time available for expiration. As a result, the mean inspiratory airflow and, consequently, inspiratory work increases. However, this strategy appears to be employed only by patients with severe expiratory air flow obstruction. End-expiratory lung volume increases during exercise in subjects with chronic obstructive pulmonary disease. This contrasts with normal subjects, in whom the end-expiratory lung volume decreases during exercise.

Exercise itself can provoke an increase of airway resistance in subjects with bronchial asthma. The exercise-induced bronchospasm is typically observed immediately postexercise. During the exercise session, an improvement in airflow is often seen. However, some subjects do develop bronchospasm during exercise. The postexercise bronchoconstriction reaches a peak during the first 15 minutes of recovery and then subsides slowly. Airway resistance may not return to preexercise levels for more than an hour. Respiratory heat and water loss appear to be the predominant mechanisms of the exercise-induced bronchospasm. The consequent hypoxemia is a result of an increased dispersion of ventilation to perfusion ratios in the lung.

Programs to improve exercise function in patients with obstructive lung disease should be designed to do the following:

- Reduce ventilatory demand, for example, administration of bronchodilators, supplemental oxygenation, pulmonary rehabilitation, and physical training.
- Improve respiratory performance, for example, bronchodilators (especially in patients who become bronchospastic during exercise), respiratory muscle training, and breathing pattern optimization.
- Reduce perception of breathing, for example, supplemental oxygen, pharmacologic, and psychogenic agents.

Patients with restrictive forms of pulmonary disease, such as diffuse interstitial fibrosis, have an increased elastic work of breathing, with a reduction of total lung capacity and its subcompartments. They respond to exercise with a rapid, shallow breathing pattern and report a high degree of dyspnea at maximum tolerable exercise. The combination of increased dispersion of ventilation to perfusion ratios and the low tidal volume leads to a high dead space to tidal volume ratio. Hyperventilation is commonly seen. Arterial hypoxemia results from both increased dispersion of ventilation to perfusion ratios and a diffusion impairment consequent to a reduced pulmonary capillary volume. These factors increase the ventilatory demand at a given work rate.

The inspiratory muscle load is abnormally high, and during exercise the ratio of tidal volume to inspiratory capacity closely approaches 1.0. The maximum exercise ventilation approaches the maximum attainable ventilation and breathing frequencies above 50 per min are quite typical. Oxygen supplementation can be used to reduce both the hypoxemia and a component of the dyspnea in restrictive lung disease, allowing an increased work capacity. However, neither the dyspnea nor the hyperventilation is abolished by this tactic.

IMPORTANT RESEARCH TOPICS

241. Establish the mechanisms of exertional dyspnea in patients with lung disease, with special reference to the interaction between pulmonary-mechanical and chemoreceptor mediation.
242. Develop improved methods of ameliorating exertional dyspnea.
243. Establish optimum training protocols to reduce the ventilatory demands of exercise and to increase the sustainable levels of ventilation.
244. Continue the search for the mechanism causing a mismatch of alveolar ventilation-to-perfusion ratios and also seek a means of reducing the mismatch.
245. Establish the contribution of deterioration of extrapulmonary systemic function (e.g., cardiovascular and muscular performance) to the impaired exercise tolerance and exertional dyspnea in patients with lung disease.
246. Determine the molecular mechanisms of exercise-induced bronchospasm and develop methods for effective prophylaxis.
247. Establish the genetic and environmental basis of obstructive and restrictive lung diseases, with the goal of preventing or alleviating the pulmonary disease.

Physical Activity, Fitness, and Kidney Diseases

The quality of life and long-term survival of patients with endstage renal disease (ESRD) are reduced, due to an accelerated development of atherosclerosis and eventual death from cardiovascular disease. The functional capacity of this population is poor. Fewer than half of the patients with endstage renal disease can increase their energy expenditure beyond the level required for walking, and most spend the majority of their time at rest. Chronic uremia, cardiovascular and musculoskeletal disease, anemia, and hypervolemia, along with poor motivation, depression, fatigue, and physical inactivity all reduce the exercise capacity of patients with chronic renal failure.

The high prevalence of hypertension, dyslipoproteinemia, reduced high density lipoprotein levels, glucose intolerance, and hyperinsulinemia accelerates atherosclerosis, causing substantial morbidity and premature mortality from cardiovascular disease in patients with endstage renal disease. This has led investigators to test the hypothesis that exercise training would improve cardiovascular function, reduce blood pressure, and improve lipid and glucose metabolism in this population.

Patients with endstage renal disease have a maximal aerobic power that is reduced on average by 50%, and a maximal heart rate that is decreased by 20 to 40 beats per minute, relative to healthy people of comparable age. Endurance training for as little as 10 weeks increased $\dot{V}O_2$max by 15 to 20% in a selected group of dialysis patients. However, training for more than six months was needed to reduce hypertension, reduce plasma triglyceride and insulin levels, raise high-density lipoprotein cholesterol, and improve glucose tolerance. Exercise training also improved muscle strength, hematological function, and psychosocial status. These changes were associated with a reduction in antihypertensive medications, and a return to employment in some exercising patients.

Multisystem involvement, severity of disease, and differences in treatment warrant that patients with endstage renal disease undergo a complete medical examination and a graded exercise test prior to exercise training. Once a stable medication, dialysis, and dietary regimen is established, compliant dialysis patients will benefit from exercise training by improving cardiovascular function, reducing risk factors for atherosclerotic cardiovascular disease, and enhancing psychosocial status and quality of life. The high risk of cardiovascular complications, increased prevalence of multiple comorbidity, frequent psychological dysfunction, and poor compliance are major factors limiting the successful conduct of exercise programs in patients with endstage renal disease. Nevertheless, there is substantial need to improve the physical health of patients with chronic renal failure, to prevent the cardiovascular complications associated with endstage renal disease, and to reduce the stress of transplantation and immunosuppressive therapy.

IMPORTANT RESEARCH TOPICS

248. Can the accelerated atherosclerosis, loss of musculoskeletal function, chronic disease, fatigue, and depression be attenuated sufficiently by exercise training to reduce medical complications and improve the quality of life in patients with chronic renal failure?

249. What are the mechanisms by which exercise (a) improves cardiovascular, metabolic, and musculoskeletal function; (b) reduces risk factors for cardiovascular disease; and (c) enhances the psychological status of patients with endstage renal disease.

250. Can early physical rehabilitation delay the progression of renal disease in patients with declining renal function by reducing metabolic, cardiovascular, musculoskeletal, hematologic and immunologic complications?

251. Are there optimal exercise regimens for uremic patients that are safe, maximize adherence, and improve both physiological function and psychological status?

252. What are the effects of erythopoietin with and without exercise on the exercise capacity and the prevalence of cardiovascular risk factors in patients with endstage renal disease?

253. Is exercise training safe and effective in improving the health and functional capacity of older patients with endstage renal disease and comorbidity, including diabetes and cardiovascular disease?

254. Multicenter longitudinal studies are needed to determine if exercise training will reduce chronic morbidity and cardiovascular complications, improve quality of life and socioeconomic status, and prolong survival in patients with endstage renal disease.

Physical Activity, Fitness, and Bladder Control

Available data on the interrelationship between physical activity, fitness, and bladder control are sparse. Lack of bladder control during physical activity is primarily a female problem, and is often caused by stress urinary incontinence. Reported prevalence rates of female incontinence vary from 8 to 52%. The large variability of results may be explained by differences in study populations, response rates, definition of the condition, and the physical activity level of the respondents. A prevalence of 33% has been shown in a gynecological practice of exercising women, and a prevalence of 26% in female physical education students.

Continence requires a higher urethral than bladder pressure (a positive closure pressure). Factors which are necessary to maintain a positive closure pressure include: (a) normal function of the central nervous system and peripheral nerves innervating the bladder, urethra, and the pelvic floor muscles; (b) normal function of the pelvic floor muscles and the smooth and striated muscles of the urethral wall to close the urethra; and (c) possibly an adequate hormonal milieu to maintain submucosal and mucosal function.

A number of risk factors for stress urinary incontinence have been identified. These include pregnancy, parity, and age. However, high prevalence rates of stress urinary incontinence have also been demonstrated in young nulliparous women.

Incontinence leads to a reduction in the sense of well-being and the quality of life, with withdrawal from physical activities, especially activities that are performed in groups. High impact activities (running and jumping) may provoke leakage in those with stress urinary incontinence. Jumping with legs in alternating abduction and adduction (jumping jacks) is the activity most likely to cause symptoms. There are no data that reveal whether chronic physical activities could cause stress urinary incontinence. Longitudinal studies would be necessary to answer this question.

Stress urinary incontinence can be treated by surgery, pharmacological agents, electro-stimulation, strength training of the pelvic floor muscles, and bladder training. On the basis of current research, it is not possible to establish the most effective form of treatment. Common problems in the studies include: uncontrolled designs; the use of different, unreliable and invalid outcome variables; inadequate assessment of pelvic floor muscle function and strength; and variations in the duration of treatment and exercise regimens.

There is no evidence that general physical activity can either prevent or treat stress urinary incontinence. However, specific pelvic floor muscle strength training is effective in 60% of women, as demonstrated in a controlled randomized study.

But over 30% of women are unable to contract the pelvic floor muscles correctly: The most common errors are the contraction of gluteal, hip adductor, or abdominal muscles or the performance of a Valsalva maneuver instead of pelvic floor muscle contractions. Most women are able to learn a correct contraction. Hence, to be effective the exercise has to be thoroughly taught. A controlled randomized study has shown that a combination of 8 to 12 maximal contractions, 3 times a day, and group exercise once a week are effective if performed for a period of at least 6 months. Pelvic floor muscle exercises should be the first choice of treatment because they are effective, noninvasive and complication-free.

IMPORTANT RESEARCH TOPICS

255. There is a need to develop reproducible and valid outcome measures of stress urinary incontinence, and methods to assess bladder and urethral function during exercise.
256. What is the normal function of the urethra and pelvic floor muscles during different forms of exercise?
257. What are the mechanisms of incontinence in nulliparous females?
258. Can strenuous exercise, such as weight lifting or marathon running, cause urinary incontinence?
259. What is the optimal mode of pelvic floor muscle exercise, the frequency of training and the duration of the exercise period when treating female stress urinary incontinence?
260. What is the mechanism through which pelvic floor muscle exercise acts to prevent and treat stress urinary incontinence?
261. Can urinary incontinence be prevented by early strength training of the pelvic floor muscles?

Physical Activity, Fitness, Immune Function, and Infection

Several infectious diseases affect highly active individuals. This may be because they perform in an environment in which certain pathogenic microorganisms are particularly widespread, or, in certain types of sport, because abrasions or other tissue injuries are likely. Highly active persons may also be at increased risk of various infections because of cross-infection from others with whom they make close contact, and from potential immunosuppression due to a combination of psychosocial stress and direct physiological effects linked to overtraining and/or participation in competitive athletic events.

Much attention has recently focused on physical and psychological stress, as potential factors modulating immune function, immune status, and upper respiratory tract infections. Because of the high incidence of upper respiratory tract infections in the general population, an understanding of the relationship between exercise and upper respiratory tract infections has potential public health implications.

The relationship between upper respiratory tract infections and exercise can apparently be modeled as a "J" curve. The risk of upper respiratory tract infections seems to decrease below that of a sedentary individual when one engages in moderate exercise training, but rises above average during periods of very heavy endurance exercise training and following exhausting endurance events.

Unusually heavy training and/or bouts of intense exercise lead to unfavorable changes in certain markers of immune function. Potential factors related to these changes may include the effects of cortisol, epinephrine, and the acute phase response to skeletal muscle damage. Several epidemiological studies have shown that risk of upper respiratory tract infections is increased in athletes following marathon-type events. Psychological stress, which alone has been shown to suppress immune function, may be a contributing factor. Regular moderate exercise training, on the other hand, may decrease the risk of acquiring an infection. Several of the immune system changes that occur during moderate exercise could improve host protection.

Various aspects of physical performance are reduced during an infectious episode. If an athlete experiences a sudden and unexplained deterioration in performance during training or competition, clinical evidence suggests that, among other possibilities, infection should be suspected. Several studies have demonstrated that exhausting exercise after contracting an infection may increase the risk of a corresponding final myocarditis. For this reason, clinicians recommend that intense exercise be restricted until full recovery.

Acquired immunodeficiency syndrome (AIDS) is a major public health problem. Questions have been raised regarding HIV transmission during sports that require close physical contact. The following recommendations regarding HIV infections in the athletic setting have taken into account earlier suggestions made by various sports medicine agencies:

- There is no evidence for HIV transmission during sports.
- Athletes infected with HIV should be allowed to participate in all sports.
- There is no justification for HIV screening prior to sports participation.
- There is a very low potential risk of transmitting HIV in some sports (e.g., boxing, wrestling).
- Each coach and trainer should receive training on the cleaning of equipment and the minimization of this risk.

Based on limited research, exercise programs for HIV-infected individuals do not appear to alter the course of disease, but may improve or preserve the individual's quality of life.

IMPORTANT RESEARCH TOPICS

262. More research is needed to improve our understanding of the threshold work rate below which exercise becomes protective and above which it is detrimental for upper respiratory tract infections.

263. Further research is warranted to elucidate the clinical significance of transient exercise-induced changes in immune status and function, and to determine which variables best predict potential changes in host protection.

264. There is also a need to examine the relation of upper respiratory tract infections in athletes and the involvement of the immune system in the tissue repair process that occurs following strenuous exercise. Could the active enmeshment of the immune system in the muscle tissue repair and inflammation process mean that protection from upper respiratory tract infections is compromised?

265. Larger, randomized, long-term, exercise training studies with HIV-infected individuals are needed to determine whether negative immune system changes can be attenuated.

Physical Activity, Fitness, and Cancer

The hypothesis that increased physical activity may be of benefit in preventing cancer development is not a new idea; the first study was reported in 1922. Early human studies (conducted up to the 1970s) yielded equivocal findings. The measurement of physical activity in these studies tended to be imprecise. Instead of measuring activity on an individual basis, investigators inferred the amount of activity from membership in a group (e.g., a specific occupation or participation in varsity sports teams). The investigators also did not consider potential confounding factors, such as body mass index and diet. Moreover, they studied only fatal cases, rather than the incidence or prevalence of the disease.

Studies of all-site cancers yielded inconsistent results. When investigators focused on site-specific cancers, the most consistent finding to emerge was an association between increased physical activity and a decreased risk of colon cancer. This observation has been consistent for both case-control and cohort study designs of varying strengths. Because cancer is a disease with a long induction period, randomized clinical trials are not feasible. Investigators studying populations from a number of developed countries have observed a protective relationship. There have been fewer studies of women than of men; nonetheless, current evidence suggests that the same relationship exists for women as for men. The protective effect of physical activity has also been documented in various ethnic groups. Although not consistently reported by all investigators, a dose-response relation appears to exist. That is, increasing amounts of physical activity appear to confer greater degrees of protection against colonic cancers. The lag time for a protective effect of physical activity remains unclear, but two studies in which physical activity during university was assessed, reported no association between such activity and the subsequent risk of colon cancer. We do not know whether different types and patterns of physical activity might offer varying degrees of protection against colon cancer. Whether certain subsites within the colon are more strongly protected by physical activity than other sites also remains unresolved. Body mass index and diet do not appear to confound, but may modify, the relationship between physical activity and the risk of developing colon cancer. A plausible mechanism for the protective relationship exists: physical activity appears to stimulate colonic peristalsis, but to

decrease segmentation. This may reduce contact between the colonic mucosa and potential carcinogens in the fecal stream, both because of the shortened transit time and because of the decrease in mixing that occurs during segmentation.

Current evidence suggests that the risk of developing rectal cancer is not associated with the level of habitual physical activity. The absence of any relationship has been shown in studies conducted in several countries, and in studies of men as well as women. The situation may differ from that associated with colon cancer, because the rectum is only intermittently filled with feces, and increased peristalsis in the large bowel may not greatly affect the duration of contact between fecal material and the rectal mucosa.

A few studies have examined the influence of physical activity on the risk of developing prostatic cancer. A protective effect, no effect, and a harmful effect of physical activity have all been reported. The biological basis for a protective relationship is plausible: high levels of testosterone may be associated with an increased risk of this cancer, and some investigators have found strenuous physical activity to decrease resting testosterone levels.

The association between physical activity and the risk of breast cancer is another area of research yielding equivocal results; two studies have reported protection and two studies of weaker design have suggested no relationship. The first study noted that physical activity protected against cancers of the female reproductive system as well. Again, a plausible mechanism for a protective relationship exists; physical activity appears to alter the gonadal hormone milieu in women, and this altered profile may reduce the risk of cancers of the breast and the reproductive system. Data pertaining to the influence of physical activity on the risk of other site-specific cancers have been scarce.

There is a paucity of data on physical fitness as it relates to all-site cancer risk. The one study of this topic reported an inverse association between physical fitness, assessed by the endurance time of a maximal treadmill test, and all-site cancer mortality. To the extent that the resting heart rate can serve as a proxy for physical fitness, one other study of three populations has reported a direct relation between resting heart rate and all-site cancer mortality, colon cancer mortality, and colon cancer incidence.

IMPORTANT RESEARCH TOPICS

266. More data are needed pertaining to the effects of physical activity on the risks

of cancer at sites other than the colorectum.

267. Once a relationship has been established for a specific cancer site, we need to address the following additional issues:

- Does the observed relationship hold for both sexes, various ethnic groups, and populations with differing lifestyles?
- At which periods of life should an individual be physically active in order to accrue any benefit?
- What types and patterns of physical activity are the most beneficial?
- Will an individual who changes from physically inactive to physically active behavior be protected against developing cancer? Conversely, will an individual who changes from an active to an inactive lifestyle lose this protection?
- Do body mass index and diet modify the relationship between physical activity and risk of the cancer?

268. Does physical activity confer uniform protection for all subsites within the colon? Or are certain subsites more strongly protected by physical activity than other sites?

269. What are the effects of physical activity in individuals who already have developed cancer?

Physical Activity, Fitness, and Recovery From Surgery or Trauma

Surgical trauma is followed by a convalescence period with decreased physical activity, decreased physical fitness, and increased feelings of fatigue extending to at least the first postoperative month. Daily physical activity (the average time spent standing and walking) is reduced in such patients during the first 6 weeks after both major and minor surgery. Those patients who are most active preoperatively also tend to be the most active in the postoperative period.

The voluntary muscle force of the elbow flexor muscles is decreased 10 to 20 days after major surgery. Measurements of handgrip force have also been made in many studies, but the results are variable. However, the response of adductor pollicis muscle to electrical stimulation is unchanged after major surgery. The oxygen uptake during standard submaximal exercise after major surgery is unchanged compared to preoperative findings. The pulse rate both at rest and during exercise is increased after surgical trauma. During identical intensities of exercise before and 20 days after surgery, the serum lactate concentration is significantly higher postoperatively. The decrease in physical activity and exercise tolerance after surgery are correlated with the postoperative decrease in body mass.

The increase in fatigue after surgery correlates with the degree of surgical trauma, the decrease in voluntary muscle force and endurance, the higher heart rate during standard submaximal bicycle exercise, and the decrease in body mass and average skinfold thickness. This increase in fatigue is independent of age and sex, preoperative anxiety, general anesthesia and duration of surgery, postoperative pain relief, and the extent of the increment in serum lactate during a standard submaximal exercise test.

Possible mechanisms to explain postoperative changes include an endocrine-metabolic response to the surgical trauma, immobilization, and decreased energy intake. A positive effect of exercise training is found after cardiac surgery, renal transplantation, and lower limb amputation. Inadequate enteral nutrition during 4 days (5 MJ/day) has no influence on either postoperative fatigue or the decrease in body mass. Intravenous nutrition during 10 days (13 MJ/day) has a positive effect on body mass and exercise tolerance postoperatively. It seems likely that the problem of recovery from surgery is multifactorial.

IMPORTANT RESEARCH TOPICS

270. What are the relative effects of epidural analgesia versus general anesthesia on physical activity and fitness after surgery?

271. What are the effects of pre- and early postoperative training on the recovery of function after surgery?

272. Does sufficient enteral nutrition influence the recovery of function?

273. Does the completeness of pain relief affect physical activity after surgery?

274. Are there interactions between analgesia or anesthesia, pre- and postsurgery

exercise training, nutrition and pain relief affecting recovery?

Physical Activity, Fitness, and Neuromuscular Disorders

The debilitating and often progressive nature of many neuromuscular diseases limits the physical activity of the affected individuals sufficiently to cause further deconditioning, which in turn accelerates their loss of functional capacity.

Individuals with neuromuscular diseases can be broadly categorized into two groups, according to whether they have apparently normal or reduced muscle mass. A lower than normal muscle mass resulting from destructive or atrophic myopathies is associated with weakness and premature fatigue; the dystrophies best represent this class of disorders. Muscle mass is more normal in disorders of muscle activation, such as myasthenia gravis, and defects of energy metabolism, such as McArdle's disease. There has been little systematic research on physical activity, training, and performance in these disorders. Nor has there been adequate assessment of the effects of exercise interventions upon the ability to undertake the activities of daily living. Information is particularly limited in those with impaired muscle activation or relaxation, and individuals with multiple sclerosis.

The maximal oxygen intake of male patients with muscular dystrophy is low, ranging from less than 15 ml/(kg $\times$ min) in Duchenne patients up to approximately 30 ml/(kg $\times$ min) in those with slowly progressive dystrophies. Submaximal exercise responses, such as the tight coupling of increases in cardiac output to increases in $\dot{V}O_2$, appear to be normal. At peak exercise, there is often a lower than expected heart rate and arterioveinous O_2 difference, the greatest deficits being associated with the most severe forms of disease and the least muscle mass. The contribution of physical inactivity to the low exercise tolerance in dystrophy has not been established. Very limited observations suggest that training may improve $\dot{V}O_2$max by 20 to 25% in some patients. However, one study reported concurrent increases in markers of muscle damage.

The muscle strength in dystrophy may range from almost nothing in end-stage Duchenne, to 70 to 80% of normal in more slowly progressive forms of dystrophy. There is often a direct relationship between strength and muscle mass, but incomplete

motor unit activation can also contribute to weakness. Case reports of exercise-induced overwork weakness, in addition to little evidence of strength gains in Duchenne patients with minimal muscle mass, suggest little or no benefit is obtained from resistance training in these patients. The best controlled studies in other classes of dystrophy, however, demonstrate large gains in dynamic and isometric strength in response to resistance training in subjects who initially possess more than 10% of the anticipated normal strength for their age and sex.

There is considerable information on exercise responses in patients with phosphofructokinase deficiency and in McArdle's disease. Such individuals can perform mild exercise effectively, but heavy exercise is associated with pain, contractures, and extreme fatigue. The $\dot{V}O_2$max of these patients is markedly reduced. In progressive exercise, the cardiac output increases much more than would be expected for a given rise in $\dot{V}O_2$.

The exercise responses of patients with disorders of lipid metabolism and of mitochondrial electron transport have also received some attention. The diverse nature of these disorders results in exercise responses that range from severely impaired to approximately normal. Data on exercise training as a potential therapeutic modality are almost nonexistent.

IMPORTANT RESEARCH TOPICS

Future research in this area of investigation must be more rigorously standardized, with larger sample sizes, most likely in multicenter trials.

275. Which patients with neuromuscular disease can benefit from endurance and resistance training in terms of their ability to undertake the activities of daily living?
276. Are conventional methods of exercise prescription appropriate for patients with neuromuscular disease?
277. What are the appropriate physiological and psychological tests to assess changes in the performance of daily activities?
278. What is the effect of endurance and resistance training on overwork weakness and muscle damage in the various forms of neuromuscular disease?

279. Can endurance or resistance training counter the deleterious effects associated with various progressive neuromuscular diseases?
280. What is the interaction among medications, exercise, and neuromuscular diseases?

Physical Activity, Fitness, and Depression

The efficacy of psychotherapy and pharmacological therapy in the treatment of depression is well documented, but it has been estimated that 21% of individuals who experience major depressive disorders are not seen in any service settings, and as many as 56% are seen by their physicians without receiving mental health services. There is also evidence that those individuals who receive treatment may not be well served. When one considers the cost and potential side-effects of antidepressant drugs, a search for nonpharmacological interventions is understandable. Psychotherapy can be particularly effective in the treatment of "non-biological" depression, and an effective adjunct when used in concert with biological interventions, but it requires a substantial investment of time and money. Finally, because of the pandemic nature of depression, neither drug therapy nor psychotherapy offers an acceptable solution. The best solution is prevention, not treatment. One potential strategy is exercise.

Exercise is associated with a decreased level of mild to moderate depression. The relationship between chronic physical activity and depression is equivocal in individuals who are not clinically depressed. However, there is limited research evidence suggesting that acute physical activity may reduce scores on depression inventories in nonclinically depressed individuals.

Excessive amounts of physical training (i.e., overtraining) increase depression scores in a dose-response manner in healthy young men and women. Severe depression requires professional treatment (e.g., medication, electroconvulsive therapy, and/or psychotherapy). The effects of exercise as an adjunct to treatment for severe depression are unclear at this time. Physically healthy people who require psychotropic medication may safely exercise if both the exercise prescription and medications are titrated under close medical supervision.

281. Is the alleviation of depression observed in clinically depressed individuals following programs of chronic physical activity caused by physical activity? If so, what is responsible for the antidepressant effect?
282. If vigorous exercise reduces depression, what mode, intensity, duration, and frequency of activity maximize this effect?
283. Since excessive exercise (overtraining) causes an adverse disturbance of mood, what is responsible for these affective changes?
284. What role does exercise play in the prevention, onset, and treatment of depression within an overall therapeutic milieu?
285. What are the acute and chronic effects of exercise on brain histochemical, biochemical, and behavioral indicators of depression?

Physical Activity, Fitness, and Anxiety

Current estimates from the U.S. suggest that 12 percent of its citizens suffer from a disruption of their "normal" lifestyle due to anxiety and anxiety-related problems. Panic attack has become the most frequent type of psychopathology. Although most anxiety disorders continue to be treated with psychotropic drugs, an increasing number of primary care physicians are routinely prescribing exercise as a treatment for anxiety. The increasing clinical awareness of the role of exercise in reducing anxiety has prompted the U.S. National Institutes of Mental Health to identify this as a topic of immediate concern.

Due to the complexity of the construct of anxiety there has not been any consistency in its measurement. Anxiety is usually recognized as a moderate to high point along the physiological arousal continuum; the individual perceives a lack of control, which manifests itself in excessive worry, fear, and heightened sympathetic arousal. This perceived lack of control eventually leads to a disruption of normal behavior patterns, with such manifestations as erratic performance and an inappropriate attentional focus.

Since increased arousal is a necessary but not a sufficient condition for the diagnosis of an anxiety response, many investigators have used physiological measures to infer anxiety. Others have focused on psychological, paper and pencil measures of anxiety. These latter measures have either been "state" measures ("how I feel right now") or "trait measures" ("how I feel in general").

At least 26 published reviews support the anxiolytic (anxiety-reducing) nature of exercise, but most reviewers caution that early studies (a) were correlational or cross-sectional in type, (b) lacked appropriate control groups, and (c) suffered from many other methodological problems (e.g., inadequate sample size, or the use of inappropriate statistical tests), thus preventing a clear interpretation of findings. Better studies dealing with the exercise-anxiety relationship are now available. A literature search ending in June, 1991, identified 148 studies on this topic, from which several conclusions may be drawn.

There is a small to moderate relationship showing that physically fit people have less trait anxiety than those who are unfit. Research designs which maximize statistical power (within subject design or optimal sample size) and have randomized group assignment are associated with larger reductions in anxiety.

When compared to untreated control groups or baseline values, state anxiety is reduced following both an acute bout of aerobic exercise and an aerobic exercise training program. The anxiolytic effects of exercise on state anxiety begin within 5 minutes after acute exercise and continue for at least 2 hours.

Reductions in state and trait anxiety are associated with activites involving continuous, rhythmic (aerobic) exercise rather than resisted, intermittent exercise. Regardless of the intensity or duration of exercise, anxiety is reduced following acute or chronic exercise. The greatest reductions in trait anxiety occur in exercise programs that continue for more than 15 weeks.

In most of the state anxiety studies, exercise has not reduced anxiety any more or less than other known anxiety-reducing treatments (e.g., relaxation, meditation, and quiet rest). Reductions in anxiety following exercise are observed irrespective of whether physiological, behavioral, or self-report measures are employed. The relationship between reductions in anxiety and increases in physical fitness is equivocal, but individuals who initially have a low level of fitness or are very anxious achieve the greatest reductions in anxiety from an exercise training program.

IMPORTANT RESEARCH TOPICS

---

286. What are the key task elements (e.g., continuous versus resisted activities, social context) which cause various exercise modes to differ in their anxiolytic effects?
287. What is the time course of the reduction in anxiety following acute exercise, and how long is anxiety reduced following an exercise program?
288. Is there a significant correlation between fitness gains with prolonged aerobic training and changes in anxiety?
289. What explanations underlie the reduction in anxiety following exercise?

Physical Activity, Fitness, and Compulsive Behavior

There has been a variety of reports of a relationship between participation in a fitness program and some sort of compulsive quality to the activity. Case studies have documented the appearance of withdrawal symptoms, self-destructive exercising because the individual cannot go without an exercise "fix," and other evidence suggesting the development of an addiction or compulsion to exercise. This negative condition contrasts with the common view that regular exercise is a positive behavior with many beneficial effects. Some attempts have been made to quantify positive and negative types of exercise participation patterns through questionnaires and interviews. Another focus of research on compulsive fitness training has been the hyperactive behavior of many eating disorder patients, particularly those with anorexia nervosa. Such individuals frequently drive themselves to exercise in a compulsive manner, usually as a means of losing weight.

High levels of physical activity are frequently noted in patients with diagnosed eating disorders, particularly anorexia nervosa. This sign appears early in the syndrome but is slow to remit. Young females who are engaged in activities which emphasize high levels of physical activity, a thin body shape, and a high level of competitiveness have a greater risk of developing eating disorders than the rest of their peer group. Some competitive athletes (predominantly female) use unhealthy and dangerous weight-loss techniques in an attempt to achieve an unrealistically low body mass. They resemble eating disorder patients in this respect, though their motivation may be enhanced performance rather than appearance. Despite the widespread belief that high levels of physical activity are associated with the personality characteristics seen in patients with eating disorders, there is no evidence to support this view.

A small subset of regular exercisers develop an unhealthy compulsion to exercise even when such exercise is harmful to their physical and mental health, social functioning and job performance. Case reports suggest that compulsive behaviors associated with exercise develop in many of these individuals.

IMPORTANT RESEARCH TOPICS

290. Research is needed on the construct validity of compulsive physical activity as distinct from an eating disorder.
291. More correlational and experimental investigations are needed to identify the factors responsible for compulsive exercising to the point of injury, social disruption, or vocational interference. There is a need to understand the prevalence and etiology of such a disorder and to determine which individuals are particularly vulnerable.
292. Research should be conducted into treatment modalities that will help compulsive exercisers return to an appropriate level of physical activity.

Physical Activity, Fitness, and Substance Misuse and Abuse

Drug abuse is an international health problem. Governments spend billions of dollars in associated health care costs, and millions of individuals experience personal tragedies and wasted lives. Even elite athletes in their prime are not exempt from risk. Thus, reducing drug abuse is a major worldwide health objective. Efforts to curtail drug abuse have to date concentrated on tactics designed to reduce supply and demand, but although controlling the supply of drugs may be helpful, officials generally agree that such approaches cannot succeed if the demand remains high. A reduction of demand is critical to prevention.

In order to prevent drug abuse through appropriate interventions, the risk factors must be known, but the causes of drug abuse are complex. Research concentrating on children and adolescents has identified a number of possible risk factors predictive of drug abuse: antisocial behavior; adverse personality traits, personal attitudes, and beliefs; family-related factors such as interpersonal relationships, parental attitudes, and behaviors; school-related factors such as academic success; peer-related factors such as the social acceptance of drugs; and genetic factors. Although many questions remain unanswered concerning the most appropriate preventive approach, one strategy which may be effective involves social learning techniques, such as the development of general coping skills through enhancement of personal and social competence. Multiple behavioral techniques may be involved, and the best opportunity currently offered appears to involve comprehensive community planning.

Physical activity and exercise may confer significant benefits relative to the prevention of drug abuse and may be an important component of a comprehensive prevention program. Such exercise-related benefits as improved mood, enhanced self-concept, increased self-confidence, and reduced symptoms of both anxiety and mild-to-moderate depression suggest that physical activity and exercise may provide a useful adjunct in alcohol and other substance abuse prevention and treatment programs.

Unequivocal evidence indicates that misuse or abuse of alcohol, cigarettes, smokeless tobacco, marijuana, cocaine, or anabolic/androgenic steroids impair health with an adverse impact on various health-related risk factors. Among participants in certain exercise and sport activities, there is an increased prevalence of substance misuse and abuse (for instance, anabolic steroids by bodybuilders and smokeless tobacco use by professional baseball players). Despite theoretical rationale and popular beliefs that exercise training may mitigate some of the adverse health risks of substance abuse, there are few data to support such a prophylactic effect.

IMPORTANT RESEARCH TOPICS

293. Can exercise training mitigate some of the adverse health effects of alcohol abuse or cigarette smoking?
294. Can certain forms of physical activity help to prevent substance misuse or abuse?
295. In those activities in which there is a higher prevalence of substance misuse and abuse, what conditions (for example, social context or task demands) predispose individuals to such behavior?
296. How useful is exercise training as a therapeutic adjunct in substance abuse treatment programs?
297. If exercise training is useful in the prevention or treatment of substance misuse or abuse, what are the underlying explanations?

Chapter 8

Physical Activity and Fitness Across the Life Cycle

The Relationship of Physical Activity to Growth, Maturation, and Fitness

Physical activity is popularly viewed as having a favorable influence on the growth, biological maturation, and physical fitness of children and youth. Inferences are based largely on comparisons of physically active and inactive individuals, and short-term experimental studies. Longitudinal studies that span childhood and adolescence and that control for physical activity are limited. Inferences about the effects of physical activity based on youngsters training regularly for specific sports have limited relevance to the general population of children and youth, since elite young athletes are a highly specialized group.

Regular physical activity has no apparent effect on statural growth and on commonly used indices of biological maturation (skeletal age, age at menarche, and age at peak height velocity). In well-nourished children and youth, these variables are primarily regulated by genetic factors. Data suggesting later menarche in female athletes are associational and retrospective, based on small samples, and do not control for other factors that influence the age at menarche.

In contrast, regular physical activity is an important factor in the regulation of body mass. Regular physical activity is often associated with a decrease in fatness in both sexes and occasionally with an increase in fat-free mass, at least in boys. Changes in fatness depend on continued activity (or restriction of energy intake) for their maintenance. Information about the possible influence of physical activity upon patterns of fat distribution in children and youth is lacking.

Regular physical activity is generally associated with greater skeletal mineralization, greater bone density, and increased bone mass. Findings are based largely on studies of experimental animals.

The effects of activity on skeletal muscle are specific to the type of training program, for example, resistance or endurance training. Metabolic responses of muscle to training in growing individuals are similar to those observed in adults, but the magnitude of the response varies. There is a lack of information on the influence of physical activity on adipose tissue metabolism and cellularity in children and youth.

Active children generally show better responses to standardized motor, strength, and aerobic power tests than inactive children. Responses to short-term training programs are generally specific to the type of program or intervention. Regular instruction and practice of motor skills result in improved motor fitness, whereas strength training programs result in significant gains in muscular strength and endurance. Training-induced increments in strength are not accompanied by increases in muscle mass in prepubertal boys. Data on responses to strength training are generally unavailable for girls. There is apparently relatively little trainability of maximal aerobic power in children under 10 years of age. It is not certain whether this observation is the consequence of low trainability, initially high levels of activity, or inadequacies of training programs. During puberty, responses to aerobic training improve considerably.

Given the limitations of cross-sectional surveys, the short-term nature of most training programs, and the lack of adequate longitudinal data that span several years during both childhood and adolescence, it is difficult to partition training- or activity-related changes from those which accompany normal growth and maturation. Training-associated changes in body composition and fitness are in the same direction as those that accompany normal growth and maturation.

Interage correlations (tracking) of fitness indicators from childhood through late adolescence are generally moderate to low, and have limited predictive utility. Tracking of fitness from adolescence to adulthood is also only moderate.

IMPORTANT RESEARCH TOPICS

298. Can growth, maturation, and fitness be differentially influenced by regular physical activity prior to and during puberty? Prospective longitudinal studies that control for physical activity and that span both the prepubertal and the pubertal years are needed.

299. Is the fitness of children more responsive to regular physical activity at certain phases of growth and maturation than others?

300. What factors influence interindividual variability in trainability during childhood and youth?

301. Is physical activity per se or fitness a better predictor of a physically active lifestyle? Should more time and effort be devoted to the assessment and encouragement of a physically active lifestyle in children and youth rather than to the assessment and development of fitness per se?

Childhood and Adolescent Physical Activity, Fitness, and Adult Risk Profile

Little information is available about relationships among children's activity and/or fitness, and their present and future health status. Such paucity of information reflects the limited validity and precision of methods that assess free-living activity during childhood; a lack of knowledge as to what constitutes "health-related" fitness in children; and limited information on the tracking of activity patterns, fitness, and associated indices of health from childhood to adulthood. Most of the current evidence is limited to cross-sectional comparisons of risk factors between active and less active (or fit and less fit) children and to short-term intervention studies.

Among otherwise healthy children, a high resting arterial blood pressure has been associated with low aerobic fitness. Exercise intervention in healthy children does not induce a reduction in blood pressure. In some, but not all studies, adiposity is more prevalent in less active children. Short-term training programs induce a mild decrease in

the percentage of body fat and, possibly, a mild increase in fat-free mass. The effect of training on the distribution of body fat is unknown. Physical activity and fitness seem to be associated with high serum high-density lipoprotein cholesterol and low serum triglyceride levels. Short-term training trials do not seem to modify the lipid or the lipoprotein profile of healthy children.

Children with chronic cardiorespiratory disease may benefit from training. This has been shown for those with asthma (exercise programs leading to a reduction in medication and possibly, a lessening of exercise-induced bronchoconstriction at a given intensity of submaximal exercise); cystic fibrosis (training programs yielding improved endurance of the respiratory muscles and an increased expulsion of mucus from the airways); and following surgery for congenital cardiac defects (where exercise tolerance and hemodynamic function are both improved by training). Short-term beneficial effects have also been shown for children with obesity (a reduction in the percentage of body fat and an improved lipoprotein profile), and for those with primary hypertension (a reduction in resting blood pressure). The long-term benefits of exercise have been studied only in children with obesity. In such individuals exercise as a single intervention has only a limited effect. Programs combining training, nutritional education, and behavioral modification may sustain weight control over several years.

The tracking of fatness, blood pressure, and lipoprotein profile from childhood to early adulthood is moderate to low, but is better from adolescence to early adulthood, particularly at the high risk limits of the distributions. Information on the tracking of physical activity patterns and attitudes toward physical activity from childhood to adulthood is inconclusive.

IMPORTANT RESEARCH TOPICS

Assuming that financial resources for pediatric exercise research are limited, preference should be given to longitudinal and interventional studies of children who already have adult risk factors for coronary artery disease, and those with family history of premature coronary artery disease.

302. What should be the "gold standard" for measuring the energy expenditure of children and youth under free-living

conditions and for assessing behavioral aspects of physical activity?

303. Are there components of fitness that are related to health status during childhood and adolescence? Which of the components, if any, that are identified in childhood and adolescence can be related to health status in adulthood?

304. What factors underlie the decline in habitual physical activity during adolescence? What are the optimal educational and/or marketing strategies to increase physical activity among teenagers?

305. How well do patterns of, and attitudes toward, physical activity track from childhood through adolescence into adulthood?

306. Is there any ethnic or racial variation in physical activity, fitness, and risk factors during childhood and adolescence? If so, what are the underlying biological and cultural factors?

307. What is the optimal multidisciplinary program to promote the long-term control of juvenile obesity?

Physical Activity, Fitness, and Female Reproductive Function

Despite high levels of fitness, many physically active women have abnormal endocrinological reproductive function. Research does not support a specific etiological role for low fatness, low body mass, hyperandrogenism, or hyperprolactinemia in exercise-associated reproductive dysfunction. This statement concerns the effects upon female reproductive function of the "stress" of exercise, mediated by neurotransmitters and hormones of the hypothalamic-pituitary-adrenal axis, and energy availability, mediated by one or more yet to be identified metabolic signals.

Abruptly imposed, prolonged, strenuous exercise training induces anestrus, ovarian atrophy, and adrenal hypertrophy in animals of several species, but such a response is not observed with more moderate regimens. Reproductive hormonal disturbances accompanying abruptly imposed strenuous exercise training but not more moderate regimens have also been reported in women. The acute release of cortisol and other "stress" hormones during intense or prolonged exercise underlies the hypothesis that activation of the hypothalamic-pituitary-adrenal axis by physical activity disrupts the ovarian axis. It is unclear, however, whether the chronically elevated levels of cortisol observed in some amenorrheic athletes are related to strenuous exercise training.

Species differences exist, but many experiments in a wide range of species demonstrate that the activation of the hypothalamic-pituitary-adrenal axis is capable of disrupting reproductive function, and that it does so during exposure to some types of stress. The stresses most commonly employed in animal studies are electrical shock and immobilization. Although these studies tend to confirm the stress hypothesis, they also raise questions about whether the exercise effects on reproductive function may be confounded by the technique used to force the animals to exercise.

The "stress" of exercise has also been confounded with an exercise-induced energy deficit in many cross-sectional and longitudinal studies of animals and humans. In many experiments, exercise and energy availability were uncontrolled. Results of some animal studies have been confounded by using food rewards to motivate the animal to exercise. Since glucose administration prevents activation of the hypothalamic-pituitary-adrenal axis during prolonged exercise, the "stress" of prolonged exercise may reflect an acute reduction in the availability of glucose as an energy source. Similar endocrine abnormalities have been reported in physically active and sedentary amenorrheic women. Therefore, the etiology of amenorrhea in physically active women may not be uniquely associated with exercise.

Anestrus has been induced by food restriction, by the concurrent administration of pharmacological inhibitors of carbohydrate and fat metabolism, by insulin administration, and by cold exposure. This would suggest that the reproductive function of mammals depends upon fuel availability. The low dietary intake and higher prevalence of reproductive dysfunction in physically active women is consistent with the hypothesis that some physically active women self-impose a chronic energy deficit, resulting in a reduced basal metabolic rate.

There is evidence to implicate both the stress of exercise and energy availability as potential etiological factors of the reproductive endocrine dysfunction observed in some highly physically active women. Carefully controlled experiments with human subjects are needed to distinguish the independent contributions of stress and energy availability and to identify the mechanisms mediating these effects.

Physical Activity, Fitness, and the Health of the Pregnant Mother and Fetus

The relationship of cardiac output to oxygen consumption and $\dot{V}O_2$max appear to be unchanged by pregnancy, whereas the submaximal oxygen consumption and respiratory quotient at a given intensity of exercise are increased. Pregnancy-related changes in stroke volume during and after exercise have not been established. Pregnant women appear to thermoregulate adequately during brief exercise in thermoneutral environments, but thermoregulation has not been studied during prolonged exertion or in different environments. The effect of quantified exercise training on measures of exercise capacity during pregnancy has also not been examined in randomized, controlled trials.

The effects of exercise on catecholamine, insulin, glucagon, cortisol, and growth hormone concentrations have been incompletely examined in mother and fetus. Further studies of mother and fetus under varied and defined exertional conditions are required, as are similar studies in patients with Type I and II diabetes mellitus and disorders of maternal blood volume and pressure.

Fetoplacental homeostasis during maternal exertion has been investigated primarily in ungulate models. In these animals, the fetal oxygen uptake is maintained despite reduced uterine perfusion, even during very strenuous acute maternal exercise. Data on fetal heart rate changes and uterine activity during brief bouts of submaximal, human, maternal exertion suggest adequate fetal homeostasis. However, maximal exertion has been followed by fetal bradycardia in some instances. The implications of this finding to fetal homeostasis under conditions of very strenuous maternal exertion are unclear. Studies of the effects of prolonged maternal exertion on transplacental fuel kinetics are limited, as are controlled studies on the effects of maternal physical training, workplace exertion, and fitness on maternal and perinatal outcomes.

The interaction of chronic exertion with maternal conditions predisposing toward fetal growth retardation (for example, chronic hypertension, cardiac disease, or chronic cigarette smoking) may be important epidemiologically. Chronic exertion may improve glucose tolerance in gestational diabetes, and may have a therapeutic role in both this disorder and Type II diabetes. Neither the chronic nor the acute effects of exertion on insulin sensitivity, glucose kinetics and metabolic rate have been examined in pregnancy.

Physical Activity, Fitness, and the Male Reproductive System

The male reproductive system consists anatomically of the hypothalamic-pituitary-testicular axis and the ejaculatory apparatus. The hypothalamic-pituitary-testicular axis is responsible for the manufacture and release of sex steroids, predominantly testosterone, and for the maturation and release of male gametes. Testicular function is controlled for the most part by luteinizing hormone and follicular stimulating hormone, both substances being released in a pulsatile fashion from the pituitary at 90-110 minute intervals, under gonadotrophin releasing hormone control. Gonadotrophin releasing hormone cannot satisfactorily be assessed in the systemic circulation, as it circulates predominantly in the pituitary portal system and has a half-life of less than 2 minutes. The pulsatile release of luteinizing hormone can be demonstrated because the luteinizing hormone half-life is 20 minutes; follicular stimulating hormone cannot usually be shown to be pulsatile, because its half-life exceeds 90 minutes. Luteinizing hormone is responsible for the manufacture of testosterone, whereas precursor availability is regulated to some degree by prolactin. Testosterone, in turn, inhibits both the production and the release of luteinizing hormone.

Testosterone is responsible for male differentiation in utero, development of secondary sexual characteristics at puberty and their maintenance during adult life. The hormone is also involved in the regulation of hepatic function, skeletal muscle growth, skeletal growth and maturation, gametogenesis in follicular stimulating hormone-primed tubules, and some behavioral aspects including sexuality. Animal data suggest that the speed of neuromuscular transmission is also affected by testosterone. Circulating testosterone is mainly bound to high-affinity, low-volume sex hormone binding globulin (~60%) and to low-affinity, high-volume albumin (~37%). The albumin-bound and free (~3%) testosterone are both biologically available.

Spermatogenesis is dependent upon testosterone and follicular stimulating hormone. The development of sperm takes up to 90 days from the initiation of gamete formation until its release into the epididymis. Full functional maturation of the sperm does not occur until after ejaculation. A peptide hormone, inhibin, is released from the testis during spermatogenesis, in turn, inhibiting both the production and the release of follicular stimulating hormone.

Short, intense bouts of exercise increase serum testosterone levels; there is debate as to what degree hemoconcentration, decreased clearance and/or increased synthesis are involved. The effects of short term exercise on serum luteinizing hormone and follicular stimulating hormone levels are unclear. It takes 20-40 minutes for a luteinizing hormone increment to induce a serum testosterone response. Because serum testosterone increments precede the time when luteinizing hormone is reported to have an effect, the testosterone increase does not involve gonadotropin stimulation of the testes.

There is a suppression of serum testosterone levels during and subsequent to more prolonged exercise and, to some extent, in the hours following intense short-term exercise. Again, the mechanisms are unclear; systems that might influence the decrease of testosterone synthesis include decreased gonadotropin, increased cortisol, changes in catecholamine or prolactin levels, and perhaps an accumulation of metabolic waste products.

Endurance training often induces a subclinical inhibition of serum testosterone levels. Changes in pulsatile luteinizing hormone release have been described, but they do not appear to be essential to the reduction of circulating testosterone levels. Clinical suppression of the hypothalamic-pituitary-testicular axis is unlikely in men. Anecdotal evidence suggests that a combination of dietary deficiencies with heavy exercise may result in decreased bone density and an increased risk of fractures. Semen quality is little affected by physical activity, with the exception of extremes of endurance training and associated weight loss. Thus, physical activity and training have measurable effects on the male reproductive system, but dietary alterations may be confounding factors. Such effects are generally physiological, and have no significant clinical consequence, except in extreme situations.

IMPORTANT RESEARCH TOPICS

316. What are the mechanisms of (a) testosterone increase with short-term exercise, (b) reduction of serum testosterone levels with acute exercise bouts of longer duration, and (c) the decrease in serum testosterone levels found with endurance training in some athletes?

317. Is there any long-term consequence of the reduced testosterone levels (both

within the accepted physiological range and more profound reductions) which are observed in some athletes?

318. What is the impact of possible interactions between training and diet on testosterone responses?

319. What are the effects of exercise and training on male fertility and sexuality?

Physical Activity, Fitness, and Aging

Aging beyond the third decade is associated with a deterioration in most physiological systems. Lifestyle changes, including alterations in physical activity and diet, and disease processes also become manifest with aging, and may contribute to the functional deterioration that is evident in older individuals. Thus, many of the deteriorations of physiological function associated with aging may result from secondary aging processes, rather than primary biological aging.

Beneficial adaptations have been demonstrated cross-sectionally in older endurance-trained athletes and longitudinally in healthy sedentary individuals up to 80 years of age who have initiated endurance exercise training. These changes typically include a reduction of body fat, increases in maximal oxygen intake and maximal cardiovascular function, decreases of blood pressure in hypertensive individuals, and possibly an increase in bone density. Endurance training generally elicits the same adaptations, at least in relative terms, in older men and women as in young and middle-aged adults. Limited data indicate that low-intensity endurance exercise training may be as, or more, beneficial than higher intensity training in the elderly in terms of compliance, adherence, reductions in blood pressure in hypertensive individuals, and minimization of the risk of injuries.

It is unclear whether changes in glucose and lipid metabolism and cardiovascular disease risk factors resulting from endurance training are an effect of exercise per se, or are due to concurrent changes in body composition. Increases in habitual physical activity may convey nutritional benefits by increasing energy expenditure and energy intake, thus leading to a larger intake of essential nutrients—protein, minerals, and vitamins—with a correspondingly reduced likelihood of developing nutritional deficiencies.

Individuals up to ages in excess of 90 years can increase their muscular mass and strength of isolated muscle groups by specific resistive exercise training. This increase in muscular strength may yield significant functional benefits for the elderly. However, it is unclear whether older individuals can increase their total body fat-free mass significantly with resistive training.

Frail, older persons generally have greatly reduced muscle mass and strength and face a host of chronic diseases that predispose them to falls and impaired mobility. The reduced physical activity normally associated with institutionalization may further exacerbate their functional impairment. Increased levels of physical activity through walking and/or strengthening exercises may reverse many of the deleterious effects of a very sedentary lifestyle.

As a consequence of diminished exercise capacity, a large and increasing number of elderly persons will be living at or just above a level of physical ability for accomplishing the normal activities of daily living. Thus, a minor intercurrent illness may be enough to render them completely dependent. An increased level of habitual physical activity may maintain or improve physiological reserves, enhancing an older individual's ability to meet daily physical demands, and thus maintaining their independence. Increasing habitual physical activity levels and exercise training are valuable interventions for the elderly, having a favorable impact on numerous factors related to their heightened rates of mortality and disability.

IMPORTANT RESEARCH TOPICS

320. Can inevitable biological aging be differentiated from secondary aging processes?

321. What are the most appropriate training prescriptions for the various modes of exercise in order to promote health, fitness, and functional capacities in different populations of older men and women?

322. What factors predispose the elderly to falls, and to what extent can improvements in strength and flexibility decrease the incidence of falls?

323. Is it possible to decrease the rate of decline in fat-free mass in very old subjects?

Chapter 9

Risks of Activity Versus Inactivity

Risk of Musculoskeletal Injuries

Among the greatest of the perceived risks of regular exercise is an increased risk in musculoskeletal injuries. Such injuries may be a deterrent to continued participation in exercise. Studies of patient groups treated in hospital emergency rooms and physician offices indicate that many persons experience musculoskeletal injury while they are engaged in either group or individual exercise and sporting activities. However, because such studies do not allow an estimation of the rates of injury in specified populations, they fail to provide information concerning the incidence of risk factors for musculoskeletal injuries during exercise participation or its absence. Such information is needed to evaluate this aspect of the cost-benefit ratio associated with being a regular exerciser.

The present statement is based on studies of adults, and because our interest is in the broad public health impact of exercise, special attention has been directed to the forms of exercise that are most prevalent in the adult population.

Some of the most commonly practiced activities in North America are, in order of decreasing prevalence, walking, gardening, running/jogging, aerobic dance, bicycling, weight lifting, and swimming. Our knowledge of the incidence of musculoskeletal injury is very limited for most of these activities. The one notable exception is distance running, for which the risk of musculoskeletal injury has been shown to be quite high (25 to 75% per year for the committed runner, depending on the manner in which injury is defined). In habitual runners the most common sites of injury are the knee and foot/ankle. Injury rates in running do not vary significantly with age or sex, but running distance and history of lower extremity injury are risk factors for injury.

Walking is generally thought to involve a minimal risk of musculoskeletal injury, but there are no studies of the incidence of injury in exercise walkers. Among competitive swimmers, shoulder injuries are relatively common, but the incidence of injuries in those who swim for exercise and physical fitness is unknown. Among aerobic dancers, the annual activity-related injury rate approximates 50%, and the risk of injury increases with the frequency of participation. Bicycling carries a significant risk of traumatic head injury and fatal bicycle accidents occur at a rate of approximately 3 to 4 per 100,000 population per year. However, little is known about the incidence of less severe musculoskeletal injuries in adults who bicycle for exercise. The risk of head trauma can be substantially reduced by wearing an effective helmet. With the other most common forms of exercise (such as weight lifting, aerobic dance, racquet sports, and softball), clinical studies have provided information on the most common types of injuries. Unfortunately, general population studies that would indicate the incidence of injury in relation to exposure are lacking for such pursuits.

IMPORTANT RESEARCH TOPICS

324. What is the incidence of musculoskeletal injury, and what are the risk factors predisposing to injury among regular participants in popular forms of exercise such as walking, aerobic dancing, gardening, and bicycling? What is the relationship between the dose of exercise and the incidence of injury? What is the effect of concurrent participation in two or more different types of physical activity on the incidence of injury?

325. Is the overall risk of musculoskeletal injury different in habitually active persons than in those who are inactive?

326. Which types and patterns of exercise optimize the ratio between the risk of musculoskeletal injury and risk of disease development?

327. What are the short- and long-term financial, behavioral, and health consequences of exercise-related injuries?

328. To what extent are "training errors" and participation in ancillary training activities like stretching and weight-training related to the risk of injury in habitual runners and participants in other activities?

Cardiovascular Risks

The cardiovascular complications of physical activity include cerebrovascular accidents, aortic dissection and rupture, cardiac arrhythmias, myocardial infarction, and sudden death. There are few data for the general population indicating the likelihood of nonfatal cardiovascular complications of exercise, and estimates of the cardiac risks of physical activity for asymptomatic persons are based largely on the likelihood of provoking sudden death. Most exercise-related sudden deaths in individuals over 30 years of age are associated with atherosclerotic coronary artery disease. However, a variety of cardiac abnormalities is associated with exercise-related deaths in young subjects.

The absolute incidence of deaths during vigorous exercise in healthy men who exercise regularly has been estimated at one death per 15,000 men per year (seven per 100,000). The hourly death rate during vigorous activity is significantly higher than that observed during less vigorous activity or when at rest. There are few studies of incidence for exercise-related sudden death in women. Available data suggest that the incidence of exercise deaths is much lower in women, undoubtedly because of the lower prevalence of coronary artery disease in middle-aged women as well as their lower participation in vigorous exercise.

There are few data on the incidence of exercise-related sudden death among young men. Available figures are often based on military personnel, who represent a selected population. For example, the exercise death rate among male U.S. Air Force recruits during basic training is approximately one per 170,000 men per year (0.6 deaths per 100,000). These results cannot be applied to the general population, because recruits are medically screened, and myocarditis appears to be more frequent in this population. The exercise-related cardiovascular death rate in Rhode Island for men under age 30 has been estimated at one per 280,000 per year (0.36 deaths per 100,000). However, the denominator for this estimate is all Rhode Island men of this age, and is not restricted to young men who exercise.

Estimates of the risk of exercise in patients with coronary artery disease are based on questionnaire data obtained from supervised cardiac rehabilitation programs. Recent results suggest that one cardiac arrest, myocardial infarction, or death occurs in every 112,000; 294,000; and 784,000 patient-hours of participation, respectively. An earlier study estimated one cardiac arrest, myocardial infarction and death per 35,000; 233,000; and 116,000 patient-hours, respectively. The lower event rates in the more recent study may be due to physicians referring healthier patients or to changes in coronary artery disease treatment.

Epidemiologic evidence continues to suggest that the cardiovascular benefits of physical activity outweigh cardiovascular risks. Such results are based on occupational and recreational exercise histories, but rarely include enough middle-aged and older subjects with extremely vigorous levels of physical exertion to calculate reliable incidence figures. Some intriguing epidemiologic results and the frequency of anecdotal reports of sudden death in vigorous exercise raise the question as to whether the risks of extremely vigorous exercise may outweigh its benefits.

Some recent reports of cardiac function following prolonged exertion suggest that the myocardium can suffer reversible dysfunction. Such studies rely exclusively on Echo Doppler-derived indices, which may be misleading. Nevertheless, they raise the question as to whether exercise induces cardiac dysfunction, whether this is deleterious, and whether this phenomenon has clinical implications in patients with ischemia or permanent left ventricular dysfunction.

IMPORTANT RESEARCH TOPICS

329. What is the pathology of, and what are the mechanisms responsible for, the possible coronary artery injuries (such as plaque rupture) associated with exercise?

330. What is the incidence of exercise-induced sudden death when determined in large populations including sufficient numbers of men, women, and children? There is also a need to establish reliable figures.

331. What are risks versus benefits of extreme exertion in middle-aged persons?

332. Are there any serious long-term consequences of repetitive exercise-induced ischemia?

333. Is the exercise induced left ventricular dysfunction suggested by Echo Doppler studies a real phenomenon and of clinical significance to healthy individuals or to patients with myocardial disease?

Chapter 10

Dose-Response Issues

Dose-Response Issues From a Biological Perspective

Any exercise that requires sustained or repeated contractions of a relatively large muscle mass activates many of the body's systems to support the process of muscle contraction. During and following exercise, local biochemical factors, along with activation of the central nervous system, stimulate the release of various hormones and affect enzymes that regulate many key metabolic functions. There are major shifts in cardiorespiratory performance, and if the activity is of sufficient intensity and duration, the renal, gastrointestinal and immune systems may become involved. Exercise also exerts physical forces on the bones, muscles, and connective tissue as a result of muscle contractions or in response to gravity. The improvement in structure, function, or health status produced by repeated bouts of exercise results from the body's immediate responses to the exercise, to the adaptations that occur over time in the body's attempt to increase its capacity or efficiency to respond to the exercise stress, or to some combination of these two responses.

The dose aspect of the dose-response relationship involves various characteristics of exercise, including type (for instance, dynamic versus static, or the amount of muscle mass used), intensity (absolute and relative to the individual's capacity), duration of session, frequency of sessions, total number of sessions, and length of time over which the sessions are performed. Other factors to be considered are baseline exercise and fitness levels, nutritional factors that might interact with exercise (for example, the intake of calcium or estrogen use may influence the effects of exercise on bone), and genetic determinants of the response. As the exercise dose that improves clinical or health status is likely to be very different from that required to improve competitive performance, it is important that the parameters of the dose-response relationship not be confined to those typically adopted when evaluating the dose-response required to improve athletic performance.

To understand the dose of exercise required to produce a specific health-related response, it would be helpful to have some idea of the nature of the mechanism of action. For example, if the response is a reduction in systemic arterial blood pressure, then to understand the dose of exercise required, it would be useful to know the mechanism by which this decrease in blood pressure is achieved. Is the lower blood pressure due to a decrease in cardiac output, a decrease in peripheral vascular resistance, or both? And what biologic changes are likely to lead to a reduction in each of these variables?

The traditional approach to the exercise dose-response issue has been to consider that the dose of exercise must produce a "training response" to be of benefit. A "training response" is a progressive change in function or structure that results from performing repeated bouts of exercise, lasts longer than hours and days, and is usually considered to be independent of a single bout of exercise. However, there is increasing evidence that some of the health-related biologic changes produced by exercise may be due more to acute biological responses during and for some time following each bout activity than to a training-induced adaptation. Examples of this type of effect include a decrease in the insulin response to a glucose challenge and an increase in lipoprotein lipase activity. If such acute changes prove to provide significant clinical benefits, then major changes may need to be made in exercise program guidelines in order to promote specific aspects of health, for example, increased frequency of activity or multiple exercise bouts per day.

Clinically significant health-related outcomes from exercise may be due to several biologic changes that have different dose-response profiles. If this is the case, then the health benefit may occur only if the characteristics of the exercise program meet the required dose (stimulus) for each of the biologic effects. A possible example of this multi-dose-response condition concerns the relationships of physical activity to decreasing the clinical manifestations of coronary heart disease. Exercise may exert its protection for heart disease through several different biological effects (changes in variables such as lipoproteins, insulin, cardiac work rate, blood pressure, and coronary artery status); each perhaps with a different dose-response profile.

Currently we know a substantial amount about the dose of exercise required to achieve many health-related physical or biological changes, but we still know very little about the optimal or minimal dose of exercise required to induce such effects in a given individual. Information on health-related biological and physical changes is still incomplete, but is adequate for the design and implementation of specific exercise program recommendations.

IMPORTANT RESEARCH TOPICS

334. What is the exercise stimulus (dose) required for a significant improvement in the various key biological changes associated with major health outcomes? How can the type, intensity, duration, frequency of exercise, and the time course of the response be defined?

335. What is the magnitude of the inter-individual variation in the dose-response relationship for the major health-related biological changes produced by exercise? Which components of the variation are due to heredity and which are due to various environmental factors? Can we identify responders and nonresponders?

336. What acute effects does exercise have upon biological outcomes that have potential health benefits? Study of this issue should consider a wide variety of exercise profiles, including prolonged low-intensity exercise as well as short bouts repeated frequently.

337. Can one discriminate between the dose-response relationship for the prevention of various pathological conditions and that needed for their treatment? For example, do the dose-response characteristics of exercise that is effective in preventing the age-related increase in arterial blood pressure differ from those lowering an already elevated blood pressure?

Dose-Response Issues From a Psychosocial Perspective

There is limited knowledge on the relationship between the dose of physical activity and the subsequent psychosocial response. Available research is frequently limited by

- the absence of a theoretical framework;
- preexperimental designs;
- weak operational definitions of the exercise dose; and
- poor external validity.

An additional problem is the meaning ascribed to the phrase "psychosocial outcomes." One can argue that these include

- overt behavior (for example, sleep and social activity);
- perception of effort (for example, the rating of perceived exertion);
- cognition (for instance, control beliefs and mental performance);
- affect (for example, anxiety and vigor); and
- the physiological outcomes of psychosocial stress.

It is erroneous to assume that the dose-response relationships will be similar for each of these different outcomes. Additionally, the concept of dose-response is in and of itself reductionistic.

The effect of a given dose of activity on any single psychosocial outcome is dependent upon subjective interpretations of the exercise stimulus (for example, the perceived intensity of exertion). Cross-sectional data suggest that the length of training influences the impact of exercise upon trait anxiety and depression. The largest effect sizes for trait anxiety are seen with programs that continue for 15 weeks or more, whereas for depression the threshold duration is 17 weeks.

Limited research suggests that reductions in blood pressure reactivity to psychosocial stress following acute bouts of aerobic exercise vary directly with exercise demands (that is, intensity and duration). In individuals with low to moderate levels of fitness, high-intensity exercise does not seem any more efficacious in influencing mood changes than low-intensity exercise.

IMPORTANT RESEARCH TOPICS

338. How does the physical and social setting of exercise influence the outcome of different doses of physical activity?

339. How are dose-response relationships influenced by subjective interpretations of the exercise stimulus and the physical and social setting of the activity program?

340. Future study of dose-response relationships should include a broad range of outcome measures, so that we might better understand the clinical implications of different doses of activity.

341. What are the interactions between dose and mode of activity with respect to psychosocial outcomes? Are there differences of response between discontinuous and continuous activities of varying intensities and durations?

342. What baseline variables modulate dose-response relationships?

Chapter 11

Other Considerations

Physical Activity, Fitness, and Quality-Adjusted Life Expectancy

Results from various epidemiological surveys suggest that adequate amounts of regular exercise will maintain or improve fitness, preserve good health, and enhance the quality of life relative to sedentary individuals. Hypertensive-metabolic-atherosclerotic disease will also be avoided or deferred, and in some studies of athletic populations, the length of life is increased. To the extent that physical activity is inadequate, physical fitness is reduced, the quality of life deteriorates, hypertensive-metabolic-atherosclerotic disease becomes more prevalent, and the risk of premature death is increased.

The important relationship between these sequences is that avoidance or correction of the undesirable activity pattern can reverse the downward path of adverse outcomes and result in a return to a more positive health status. An inactive individual may become physically more active, an unfit person may regain fitness, the risk of hypertensive-metabolic-atherosclerotic disease can be reduced, and life becomes longer, healthier, and more satisfying; all these follow if physical activity is adequate and maintained over the life span.

Factors other than physical activity such as inheritance, infection, nutrition, injury, environmental, and situational circumstances can all intervene and either promote or detract from the good quality, prolonged life to which the individual aspires. Yet, the past decade has seen wide acceptance of evidence that adequate levels of leisure-time physical activity promote health-related fitness and positively influence health status, quality of life, and longevity, even though the requirements for promoting these advantages in the individual and on a population are not fully defined.

One study of male United States university alumni aged 45 to 84 years, followed from 1977 to 1985, has indicated that lower all-cause death rates accompany an increase in the vigor and frequency of walking, stairclimbing, sportsplaying, and physical activity in general. The lower death rates are also accompanied by lower levels of cigarette smoking, and a lower body mass index, and by normotensive and euglycemic status, but show little association with a history of prolonged parental survival. Sedentary men (leisure energy expenditure <8 MJ/week), who contributed 58% of the man-years in this particular study, were at 19 to 66% (95% confidence intervals) greater risk of mortality during the nine-year follow-up period than more active men. Cigarette smokers showed 54 to 127% added risk over nonsmokers. Hypertensives had a 28 to 76% higher risk than normotensives. The more obese individuals were at 0 to 40% greater risk than men who were more lean. However, a background of early death in one or both parents added little to the risk of premature mortality (−9 to 20%).

Eleven to 15 years after the initial assessment, 23% of the men had remained active, 16% had converted from physically active to a sedentary status (leisure energy expenditure <8 MJ/week), 19% had converted from sedentary status to physically active, and 42% continued to be sedentary. Men who had increased their physical activity reduced their risk of death from 5 to 42% relative to those who now exercised less. Men who had decreased their physical activity level (often times because of chronic illness) increased their risk of death only slightly (−10 to 56%) versus those who had continued sedentary. Men who took up moderate sportsplay, versus those who continued to avoid it, reduced their risk between 14 and 43%. Other lifestyle factors were also associated with longevity. Men who quit smoking reduced their death risk by 8 to 43%. Long-term hypertensives were at greater risk of death than those more recently reported hypertensive. Maintenance of a lean body mass had survival advantages over continued obesity, becoming obese, or losing weight from a previously obese status.

These findings for males aged 45 to 84 years translate into estimates of extended survival when subjects are followed through to a maximum age of 85 (85 years being the approximate male lifespan). Changed lifestyles added years totalling: 0.24 to 1.30 years, for increasing physical activity to adequate level; 0.55 to 1.61 years, for taking up moderate sports; and 0.25 to 1.83 years, for quitting cigarettes. Even among the elderly, the combination of adding moderate sportsplay and stopping the smoking habit yielded a substantial gain in longevity (for example, 1.62 years for men aged 65 to 74 years, and 0.63 years for those aged 75 to 84 years).

The men who took up a more active lifestyle between the 1960s and 1977 not only increased longevity, but also reported improvements in health. They were more likely to report that they "felt younger than their years" and that they "felt fine and enjoyed life" than were those who had remained sedentary. The men who became more active were also less likely to develop cardiovascular and metabolic disorders during the nine-year follow-up.

IMPORTANT RESEARCH TOPICS

---

343. How much, what kinds, how intense, and for whom should physical activity be prescribed in order to improve and/ or maintain health (physical, psychological, social, cultural, and spiritual well-being)?
344. How much short- and long-term physical activity is needed to induce an optimal level of physiological fitness, that is, a functional integration of all body systems?
345. How can longevity be extended to its optimum, that is, with preservation and enhancement of high quality living?
346. How can physical activity, health-related fitness, dietary and other lifestyle habits, environmental circumstances, and heredity best be integrated in our search for optimal health?

Costs and Benefits of an Active Versus an Inactive Society

Can corporate or national health care costs be reduced by increasing the prevalence of regular exercise? By extension, is the cost of achieving any improvement in health that results from greater exercise offset by a reduction in the costs of medical services? Because an increasing share of individual health care costs are borne by company-funded employee insurance programs in the United States, recent studies in that country have focused on the individual as a member of a work site employee group. In other industrialized countries, most of which have public health insurance, there is also concern about rising medical costs. Sometimes the work site has been adopted as the unit of analysis, and other studies have examined the impact of physical activity upon the population. In the private sector, a further motivation for offering exercise programs has been to enhance productivity.

Several investigators have sought to determine whether the physically active employee or member of the community is more productive, is less frequently absent from work, is injured less often, changes employment less frequently, and has a higher morale than a more sedentary person. A number of studies show potentially beneficial associations between physical activity and these variables. Correlations are generally statistically significant, but the strength of these relationships is generally low, leaving decision-makers with a good deal of uncertainty regarding the cost-benefit ratio for programs designed to enhance employee or community fitness.

A more global concern, of special importance to health economists, is the impact of improved health on longevity, and hence, on the burden that might be imposed upon company-sponsored and/ or national medical and pension benefits by longer-living retirees. If improved worker health, as an outcome of increased physical activity, is translated into increased longevity (and total medical care costs for these retirees per year of life were to stay the same), such an outcome could be viewed as a liability to society and to the former employer. However, there is some suggestive evidence that active individuals will develop less chronic disease in their later years, and will die without incurring the costly extended final illness seen in many sedentary people. A longer lifespan not only has a potential impact upon medical costs, but also implies a longer total period of pension distribution, if the age of retirement also remains constant. Again, this potential cost would be offset if the retirement of a healthier person were delayed to a more advanced age. The current trend seems to be in the opposite direction, as improved pension and investment income programs support earlier retirement, although it is unclear how far accumulating medical problems influence an individual's decision to take premature retirement.

Unlike biological studies of the effects of enhanced physical activity, cost-benefit questions are frequently studied in the context of a quasi-experimental research design. In a recent evaluation of over 400 published reports of health promotion program outcomes, the vast majority were deemed insufficiently well controlled to draw firm conclusions, let alone to establish causal relationships. Given the paucity of firm, well-controlled research, some proponents of corporate and community fitness programs have prematurely advanced conclusions regarding the economic benefits of such programs. In fact, poorly supported claims detract from the probable positive outcomes that may ultimately be demonstrated. But, even if no positive return on investment is eventually concluded from more sophisticated research, good health as an outcome of increased physical activity may be its own inherent return. In other words, cost-effectiveness may be demonstrated even in the absence of a favorable cost-benefit ratio defined in strict monetary terms.

IMPORTANT RESEARCH TOPICS

347. The economic impact of exercise on the individual and on society remains unanswered, due principally to the difficulty of measuring change in a poorly controlled experimental environment. One approach has been to develop computer simulation projections of costs and benefits based on normative population data, with sensitivity analyses included as an essential part of such studies. However, such initiatives await stronger input data from well-controlled randomized trials.

348. Another issue to be resolved is the lack of standardized program elements, definitions, and descriptions of outcomes. Standardization of these various terms must be achieved to allow comparisons between studies.

349. What elements comprise an acceptable corporate or community program? How is the outcome modified if other lifestyle modules such as smoking cessation are added? How should medical costs be defined: direct costs or total costs? What are the social costs and benefits of extended survival? How can productivity, absenteeism and turnover be measured accurately?

350. Since the quantification of psychological and behavioral outcomes (such as improved morale and greater productivity) are currently an uncertain science, should research focus on program cost-effectiveness rather than on cost-benefit analysis?

351. How does cost-effectiveness differ between the work site programs in manufacturing and insurance companies which have been most often studied to other industry and community settings; for instance from white salaried employee groups to minority and hourly-rate groups, and from large organizations to employees from smaller companies.

352. Would cost-effectiveness ratios differ for those who are currently inactive? What is the marginal return on such investment?

353. Most work site studies have concentrated on in-house employee programs with well-developed facilities. Many corporate programs, especially for smaller companies, have purchased memberships in commercial or community programs such as the YMCA. What are the cost-benefit ratios and the cost effectiveness for such arrangements?

Heredity, Activity Level, Fitness, and Health

Interindividual differences in the base sequence of DNA are the source of human genetic variation. Each human being has about one variable DNA base for every 100 to 300 bases, so that each one of us is genetically unique. Inherited differences are likely to be involved in determining the health status of a person as well as the interrelationships between individual components of the physical activity-fitness-health paradigm.

The contribution of genetic factors to interindividual differences in the level of habitual physical activity has not been extensively studied, but available data suggest that it accounts for about 30% of the phenotypic variation. The evidence that heredity is involved in determining interindividual variability in health-related fitness is more abundant, although the quality of the evidence varies according to the component considered and the methods that have been used to estimate heritability. Most of the data are from twin studies; heritability estimates derived exclusively from twin data are generally higher than those based on family data or relatives by adoption, and often vary quite widely from one study to another. Significant genetic effects have been reported for most factors associated with morphological fitness, with typical values ranging from about 25% for total body fat content to 30 to 50% for regional fat distribution phenotypes. Such effects are presumably polygenic, but major gene effects have also been reported to contribute to the variation in body mass index and some regional fat distribution phenotypes. Heritability estimates of various muscular and motor fitness phenotypes are largely derived from twin data and are generally well over 50%. The use of a wide range of tests to assess this component of fitness has contributed to the highly heterogeneous heritabilities reported in the literature.

Among the components of cardiorespiratory fitness, blood pressure is the variable that has been most studied by geneticists; heredity accounts for about 30% of interindividual differences in resting blood pressure. The contribution of heredity to submaximal exercise capacity and maximal aerobic power reaches about 20 to 30% of the phenotypic variance. More studies are needed to assess the genetic contribution to cardiac and pulmonary functions. Because of its association with common familial diseases like diabetes and cardiovascular disease, several components of metabolic fitness have been studied extensively; for instance, heritability levels reaching about 50% of the age- and sex-adjusted phenotypic variance for plasma triglycerides, total cholesterol, and the various lipoprotein fractions have been commonly reported.

The genetic factors responsible for interindividual differences in health-related fitness do not operate in a vacuum, but are constantly interacting with lifestyle and personal characteristics, as well as with the social and physical environment. Therefore, genetic factors may influence the response of phenotypes to environmental stimuli like regular physical activity. There is now good evidence that the extent of the response of health-related fitness factors to regular physical activity or dietary intervention is strongly determined by unknown genetic characteristics. Inherited differences appear to be more important in determining the adaptive response to regular physical activity than in determining the absolute initial level of the health-related phenotypes.

IMPORTANT RESEARCH TOPICS

354. We need to identify the genes that contribute to interindividual differences in each health-related fitness phenotype.
355. We need to determine the impact of allelic variation at relevant genes on (a) the level of health-related fitness phenotypes, (b) the response of these phenotypes to regular physical activity, and (c) the covariation between these health-related fitness phenotypes. An important question is whether the genes associated with individual differences in the response to regular exercise are the same for each health-related fitness component.

Physical Activity and Fitness: Evolutionary Perspectives and Trends for the Future

On our approximately 4.6 billion-year old planet, the first forms of life are estimated to have appeared some 3.5 billion years ago. Two billion years later, the unicellular living organism with a nucleus had evolved. The fundamental biological principles that sustain life were developed by a process of natural selection. If a comprehensive textbook of biochemistry had been written 1.5 billion years ago, it would no doubt be up-to-date in its treatment of cell function. Processes such as the breakdown and resynthesis of ATP, PCr, glycolysis, and aerobic energy production via the Krebs citric cycle and the respiratory chain were already well-developed. Evolution was now ready for its next major step, the emergence of larger animals, an era which began some 700 million years ago. Mammals are represented during the last 220 million years of the process, and the first primates entered the scene some 120 million years ago.

African fossils reveal the presence of a hominid *Australopithecus* about 4 million years ago. Several species of this genus survived for several million years, and one was the ancestor of the genus Homo, *Homo habilis*, about 2 million years ago. The species *Homo sapiens* (modern man) has probably existed for at least 40,000 years to date. The transition from the lifestyle of a roaming hunter and food gatherer to the less mobile farmer began some

10,000 years ago. Technological developments during the last 100 years have introduced a rate of change far exceeding all that occurred during the preceding 4 million years of hominid evolution.

A consequence of these changes in lifestyle is that humans have participated in gigantic experiments without any control groups. Our ancestors lived in small bands of perhaps 15-30 individuals as a cooperative society "in which individuals and environments continuously interrelate and affect each other." An individual's age was not measured in years, but rather in terms of accumulated experience. Education began when a child had matured enough to understand the messages of his or her teacher. Thus, the boys learned from the "retired" hunter, who had entered a new niche in society, carrying out a task that was still intellectually and physically demanding and of vital importance to the future of the group. There were no well-defined relationships between socio-occupational roles and a person's age in that era!

Many expressions of human behavior, which were very appropriate adaptations to life in small bands, would be close to "catastrophic" if adopted by large and modern societies. Despite the currently expressed desire of some indigenous populations, there seems no way that humans could revert to their historic "natural" way of life. But with adequate insight into our biological heritage, we may be able to modify our current, partly self-destructive lifestyle. The human body has adapted to the needs of regular, moderate physical activity, and a continuation of such activity is essential for its optimal functioning. This volume illustrates the many scientific efforts to study the value of restoring an active lifestyle as a tactic for the primary and secondary prevention of various disorders and diseases. In the future, the early study of DNA sequences may allow us to determine individuals who are at a particularly high risk of morbidity and mortality from specific diseases. It may then be possible to develop and implement preventive programs adapted to the needs of those individuals. Will it also be possible to predict a person's response to a given training program or to a change in diet from a review of blood lipids, blood pressure, maximal aerobic power, muscle strength, endurance, and the like? To take an extreme viewpoint: do those involved in health promotion have the right to "manipulate" the lifestyle of 100 persons in order to save three lives, particularly if the remaining 97 people neither enjoy nor need the exercise program but are also strongly encouraged or even "forced" to participate? At present, we are unable to predict which three individuals would

benefit from a more active lifestyle. But what about in the future?

The United States Census Bureau has estimated that the proportion of Americans who are older than 65 years will double from 12% of the population in 1986 to 24% in 2020. Other developed and developing societies face similar challenges. Current gerontological research has emphasized the average age-related losses of function and has neglected to consider the substantial heterogeneity of older persons, which is in part a consequence of activity history and in part a consequence of genetic individuality. The functional effects of the inherent aging process have, in consequence, been exaggerated, and the modifying effects of diet, physical activity, personal habits, and psychological factors have all been underestimated. Within the category of normal aging, a distinction should be drawn between "usual aging," in which extrinsic factors heighten the inevitable, inherent effects of aging, and "successful aging," in which extrinsic factors play a neutral or a positive role. Aging is necessarily associated with some reduction of maximal aerobic power and muscle strength, but the functional ability of an active 65-year-old Canadian exceeds that of a sedentary young adult. Being overweight is an additional handicap at any age. In combination with the other changes seen in the frail elderly, it makes walking, climbing stairs, getting up from a bed or a chair, or entering a bus or a train more difficult, fatiguing, and eventually impossible. Aging persons thus lose their independence and autonomy. As a consequence of a progressive loss of functional capacity, large and increasing numbers of elderly persons live below, at, or just above the "thresholds" of physical ability needed for independence. A minor intercurrent illness is then sufficient to make them completely dependent.

In the United States, the life expectancy at birth has increased from an average of 47 years in 1900 to approximately 75 years in 1988, and in other countries the average expectancy is now substantially greater than this. What are the upper limits to average human longevity? It has been calculated that if ischemic heart disease were to be eliminated, the life expectancy at birth would increase by 3.0 years for females and 3.5 years for males. If all forms of cancer (22.5% of all deaths in 1985) were also eliminated, life expectancy would increase by 7.0 years for females and 8.1 years for males. In other words, elimination of these two major categories of disease would not lead to any dramatic increase in life expectancy. Technological advances in terminal medical treatment rather than a reduction in the prevalence of risk factors for chronic disease have allowed frail elderly persons who are suffering from fatal degenerative diseases to survive longer after the onset of disease than was the case in the past. Research efforts by the medical community have focused on prolonging the duration of life rather than on preserving its quality. The time has come to shift the emphasis of research toward preserving and ameliorating function in people with the nonfatal diseases of aging. One sad but important factor is ethical, including human and legal aspects of euthanasia in seemingly hopeless cases.

In this bizarre world, we notice overfeeding and the negative effects of a sedentary lifestyle in developed countries, but do little to help the millions of people who are living under marginal or very poor conditions in the "Third World." It is impossible to follow the advice to exercise and be active in societies where there is not enough food to cover even the energy demands of basal metabolism. This planet produces more food than its population needs, but it is poorly and inequitably distributed. Medical advances, including mass vaccinations, allow more and more children to survive in "Third World" countries, but what quality of life

will they face as they become adults? Life has always been complicated: if we transform hominid history over a 4-million-year period into a 400 m race, it has become more complicated during the last meter (10,000 years) and particularly during the last 10 mm (100 years).

We must take a global view, and not "forget" the urgent health needs of the "Third World." However, priority one of the health scientist, from a realistic viewpoint, is to concentrate on health promotion in the developed countries. Open-air recreational activities are an effective source of physical activity that is well anchored in our biological heritage. Education in "fauna and flora" was once essential to survival. Similar education today is unfortunately neglected, but it could create an excellent lifelong, hobby interest. There are those who do not like walking just for the sake of walking, but if a hobby like bird-watching demands some walking, they will be prepared to walk. And family members, neighbors, or even business associates can also go out to "walk and talk." The message of enhanced physical activity will seem more practicable and realistic when we find such ways to incorporate regular exercise into our daily living.

Additional books from the 1992 International Conference on Physical Activity, Fitness, and Health

Physical Activity, Fitness, and Health

Projected to be available in late 1993

For those who want more in-depth information than is provided in *Physical Activity, Fitness, and Health Consensus Statement*, this volume includes the entire proceedings from the 1992 International Consensus Symposium on Physical Activity, Fitness, and Health. In addition to the consensus statement that summarizes the latest knowledge in the field, it includes over 70 supporting papers written by world-renowned exercise scientists who analyze the state of research in their areas of expertise. Projected to be more than 1,000 pages, it is a storehouse of authoritative information for exercise scientists and researchers.

Active Living

Projected to be available in late 1993

Practitioners, instructors, and students who want a concise and accurate look at the scientific knowledge on physical activity, fitness, and health will want this collection of papers from the 1992 Active Living portion of the 1992 International Conference on Physical Activity, Fitness, and Health. It features 42 papers that concentrate on how practitioners can use the current base of knowledge in the physical sciences to help them in their day-to-day work.

If you would like to receive further details on these forthcoming titles, please contact Human Kinetics Publishers and we'll send you complete descriptions and ordering information as soon as it becomes available.

Human Kinetics Publishers
Box 5076
Champaign, IL 61825-5076
USA

Toll free: (800) 747-4457
Telephone: (217) 351-5076
Facsimile: (217) 351-1549

Human Kinetics Publishers (Canada)
Box 2503
Windsor, Ontario N8Y 4S2
CANADA

Toll free: (800) 465-7301
Telephone: (519) 944-7774
Facsimile: (519) 944-7614

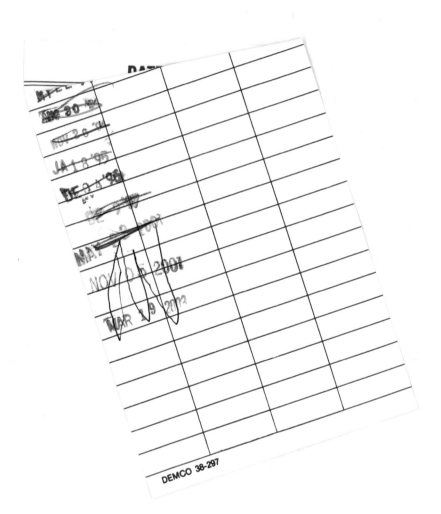